WHAT HURTS THE PHYSICIAN HURTS THE PATIENT

MedRAP: A Comprehensive Approach
to Improving Physician Training,
Professional Development and Well-Being

IRIS MUSHIN, M.ED., MBA

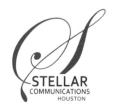

STELLAR
COMMUNICATIONS
HOUSTON

WHAT HURTS THE PHYSICIAN HURTS THE PATIENT
MEDRAP: A COMPREHENSIVE APPROACH TO IMPROVING PHYSICIAN
TRAINING, PROFESSIONAL DEVELOPMENT AND WELL-BEING

NOTICE AND DISCLAIMER

This textbook has been written for use in connection with education of medical professionals in matters relating to professional development, including organizational and communication skills. This textbook is not intended for reference use as a medical or scientific treatise and should not be used or relied upon in any manner as authority for any standard of care or for purposes of diagnosis or treatment of any medical condition. Material and information referenced herein relating to specific medical conditions, including without limitation, matters relating to medical procedures, or prescription or use of any drug, is included exclusively for illustrative purposes in order to identify commonly encountered conditions, problems, and issues to be addressed by the professionals implementing the curriculum.

Neither the author nor the publisher provides any representation or warranty, express or implied, as to the accuracy or completeness of the information provided in this textbook. Neither the author nor the publisher shall have any liability to any person for any damages, whether physical, psychological, emotional, financial, consequential, special, incidental, or for any punitive or exemplary damages, arising from use or misuse of this textbook.

For information, contact Stellar Communications Houston.
Published in the United States of America.

Paperback ISBN: 9781944952174
E-book ISBN: 978-1-944952-18-1
Library of Congress Control Number: 2018938706

Published by Stellar Communications Houston LLC
www.stellarwriter.com
281.804.7089

*To my husband, who was my inspiration and greatest supporter for this book,
and to my children, with much love and gratitude.*

CONTENTS

FOREWORD

WHAT HURTS THE PHYSICIAN HURTS THE PATIENT IS THE RESULT OF A CAREER'S work and a labor of love by Ms. Iris Mushin. Ms. Mushin approached Dr. Edward Lynch, the program director of Internal Medicine, and me, while I was serving as Chair of Internal Medicine at Baylor College of Medicine in 1989, requesting our support to carry out a pilot program aimed at improving the internal medicine residency program at Baylor College of Medicine.

The ultimate goal was to develop a resident assistance program, RAP, for the Internal Medicine Department of Baylor College of Medicine. The pilot project was a success, and 28 years later, Ms. Mushin has produced a wonderful publication describing MedRAP: a Medical Resident Assistance Program, that addresses training, professional development, and the well-being of Internal Medicine residents. At the time she initiated the project, Ms. Mushin was an MBA student, and she subsequently directed the program over the next two decades; she made an enormous contribution not only to resident training at Baylor, but also to the overall training of residents in the United States.

As a way of background, at the time when Ms. Mushin undertook this project, the burnout rate was 63% in internal medicine, one of the highest of the medical specialties. This was at a time before the adoption of the "Libby Zion rule" that limited the resident work hours to 80 hours a week. At the time, residents often worked as long as 120 hours a week. Not only has the MedRAP program contributed to improving the training and lifestyles of medical residents, it has also paved the way for activities such as competency evaluations, which are now mandatory for the accreditation of residency programs.

Ms. Mushin's publication is comprehensive, clearly written, and will be of enormous value to all individuals, trainees, administrators, and directors of medical residency programs. Many of the chapters deal with activities which have now become commercialized: for example, there are now software programs for tracking residency activities and for assuring maintenance of criteria for accreditation. This is an excellent contribution and reflects very positively not only on the author, but also on Baylor College of Medicine, and its support of the MedRAP training program for many decades.

I highly recommend this book to all medical residents, resident program directors, department chairs, and administrators who are connected with the training of new physicians.

Antonio Gotto, Jr., MD, DPhil.
Dean Emeritus, Weill Cornell Medicine
Provost for Medical Affairs Emeritus, Cornell University
December, 2017

A PROGRAM DIRECTOR'S PERSPECTIVE ON MEDRAP

As a resident in the internal medicine residency program at Baylor College of Medicine when there was no MedRAP program, and subsequently as the Program Director of that same residency program after MedRAP had been operational for nearly a decade, I have witnessed the benefits such a program offers on multiple levels including that of individual residents, the training program, and the institution as a whole.

MedRAP significantly improved resident morale and helped develop leadership skills as part of the training program. Both one-off and systemic problems were more quickly identified, and the accelerated flow of information to management of the residency program and hospitals, coupled with potential solutions identified within the MedRAP process, resulted in more rapid implementation of many improvements.

The annual structured hospital-specific Quality Improvement component taught trainees useful skills, but also became an integral part of the Residency Program's efforts to improve education and patient care at the teaching hospitals. Moreover, as residency education and its oversight by the ACGME has evolved, the MedRAP program helped facilitate ACGME compliance across multiple domains.

Importantly, in this era of increasingly limited resources and cost constraints, the cost of the entire MedRAP program was nominal in comparison to the significant return on investment it delivered. Indeed, I would argue that the importance of resident education coupled with the costs, both financial and otherwise, of a dysfunctional program or ACGME non-compliance, means that for many programs, not instituting a program such as MedRAP is actually the more expensive decision.

The bottom line is that a program such as MedRAP benefits training programs and medical institutions as it provides a cost-effective platform for improving the Graduate Medical Education experience for trainees, faculty, other healthcare professionals, and patients. I highly recommend not only reading this book, but also implementing its lessons at your training program.

Amir Halevy M.D., J.D.
Director, Internal Medicine Residency Program, 2000-2006

PREFACE

THE "BUTTERFLY EFFECT" DESCRIBES HOW VERY SMALL CHANGES IN A COMPLEX system can produce results that may have a significant impact. The term refers to the idea that the mere beating of a butterfly's wings produces minor atmospheric variations that may ultimately alter the path of a storm, delay or accelerate its course, or even prevent it altogether. What might seem an insignificant change in one location can result in progressively larger differences somewhere else or at a later stage. In an organizational context, the Butterfly Effect posits that any decision we make now, no matter how small, can play an essential role in bringing future changes to organizations.

The Medical Resident Assistance Program (MedRAP) described in this book was developed to facilitate the transition of young physicians from medical school to residency and to improve their professional development and training environment. Just as the Butterfly Effect can result in progressive changes, the implementation of this program produced gradual changes that helped transform the organizational culture in the training program and had a beneficial effect on the medical residents, the department, and its four affiliated hospitals.

I conceived the idea for this program in 1988, when my husband was completing his surgical training at Baylor College of Medicine and I was studying for my MBA. As the wife of a surgical resident, I already understood the stress of medical training, having experienced it on a very personal level. I was prepared for my husband to endure hard work and long hours—residents often worked 120 hours a week, were frequently on call, and got very few days off. However, life for the residents was even more taxing than I had anticipated. I was not prepared for the difficult and negative training environment I witnessed or the recurring lack of respect my husband and the other medical trainees experienced.

Negative treatment by members of the health care team was a frequent occurrence for which there was little recourse or remedy. I saw my husband and his colleagues work long hours with dwindling physical and emotional energy. Over the course of that year, I came across many residents and fellows who were struggling personally and professionally, culminating in depression, burnout, divorce, and even suicide attempts.

At the time, there were no requirements for residency programs to address work hours, professional issues, or the general well-being of graduate medical education (GME) trainees. When I sought information about support mechanisms for the medical residents, I discovered that the staff psychiatrists were inundated with calls from residents and that the existing stress-management programs were considered ineffective by many of these young physicians.

Discovering this lack of support, I decided to explore these issues further. I found a troubling correlation between the negative training environment and less-than-optimal patient care. I began to see how it might be hard for residents to have compassion for their patients in an environment that had no compassion for them. This was not just an issue of training or life quality; it was a public health issue that was not being addressed, and it was adversely affecting patient care. Unfortunately, very little was being done to connect the dots between the residents' training environment and quality of care.

At the time, GME provided solutions that treated the symptoms rather than the causes. To counteract the harmful effects of stress, residents were encouraged to exercise more and attend meditation workshops using techniques such as Dr. Benson's "Relaxation Response." In other cases, residents were referred to mental health professionals for assistance. However, in the context of 120-hour weeks, hazing by some of the health care team members, and the unrelenting demands of patient care on young physicians with no clinical experience, meditation and psychotherapy were not enough.

As an MBA grad student with an interest in organizational systems, I began to examine my husband's experiences in various hospital rotations to understand how his training could be improved. Problems in the medical training environment were contributing to widespread burnout and dissatisfaction among residents. The issues contributing to a negative work environment were systemic: the same types of problems were repeated with each new group of incoming residents, and over time, these patterns became ingrained within the culture of these hospitals where graduates were employed as attending physicians.

While in business school, I was exposed to a number of organizational concepts from various industries. These methods were developed to facilitate the transition of new employees into their respective roles. I began exploring the possibility of applying these principles to residency training programs. I approached two leaders at Baylor College of Medicine (the program director and the chair of the Department of Internal Medicine) with the idea of creating a program to address the issues.

I developed a pilot study, drawing on my training in management education and psychology, to explore the idea of improving the residency experience by utilizing organizational theory approaches to help alleviate the stress residents were experiencing. The program started with a needs analysis to assess the challenges that medical residents faced and identify ways to ameliorate them. The problems identified were systematically analyzed before any conclusions were drawn, which increased the likelihood of developing programs structured to deal with real, rather than assumed, needs. The results of the needs analysis highlighted several primary areas of concern.

The first finding was the need for a place where residents could provide confidential feedback. The feedback in the formal departmental evaluations was different from the feedback I received directly from the residents during confidential interviews. In the formal evaluations, residents communicated only mundane concerns related to training and the hospital environment. However, in confidential interviews, residents expressed great distress and dissatisfaction with their training and with inefficiencies in patient care in the affiliated hospitals. This discrepancy confirmed that residents were reluctant to provide feedback to their superiors about the difficulties they experienced in their training and in clinical environments. Important information was not being communicated to those in charge of managing the program. This was not in the best interest of the residents, the residency program, the hospitals, or the patients.

The second finding was inconsistent mentorship. The first-year residents' experience and subsequent performance varied wildly depending on the skills of the senior residents who were team leaders. Some senior residents were more helpful than others, which impacted the performance of the junior residents, especially while on hospital ward teams. The attitude and skills of the senior resident team leaders directly affected the residents' experience. There was a need for additional opportunities for developing positive mentorship relationships with senior residents who were viewed to be helpful, effective, and professional.

The third finding was the lack of any effective mechanism for senior residents to share the knowledge they had acquired over the years, as well as their experiences dealing with the many challenges they encountered in the early years of their residency. The collective wisdom of past generations was not effectively communicated to the PGY-1 (Post Graduate Level 1) residents; thus, they were often left to re-invent the wheel, not always with the best results and sometimes at the expense of patients and their families. There was a need to formalize and streamline the informal training that was, until then, provided randomly without any structure.

Based on the results of the pilot study and the findings of the needs analysis, the program was fully implemented and made available to all incoming residents the following academic year.

MedRAP ran successfully for 25 years at Baylor College of Medicine. Throughout those years, I received numerous cards and letters from residents and fellows, thanking me for establishing the program and helping them through residency. One resident's message, in particular, has stayed with me:

"Have you ever attended a ceremony where the act of candle lighting took place? A single candle is lit; it lights another, and then another, and so on until a whole circle of candles are lit. As it is with a single candle, so it is with a single person. Your program touched others with its light, and lives were changed through an endless chain of human contacts. Working with you these past few months has been invaluable to me..... Thank you."

It was the power of the supportive community that nurtured the growth of these young physicians.

Over the years, MedRAP has helped hundreds of resident participants who have gone on to become faculty, program directors and chairs in academic institutions all over the U.S. Hopefully, the strategies they acquired during the program continue to impact the learning environments in other institutions.

Today, the Accreditation Committee for Graduate Medical Education (ACGME) has set work-hour limits for residents and established standards to enhance residents' education. Competencies are assessed in areas such as professionalism, interpersonal communication skills, and ability to improve the hospital system and patient care. Thus, the resident training experience is much improved. Training programs are evaluated and accredited based on their success in meeting the ACGME competencies. However, new challenges are emerging, such as dealing with time pressures and changing regulations. Some old challenges and stressors still lead to unnecessary stress and burnout, both of which have been reported to increase even after the implementation of limits on work hours. The well-being of young doctors continues to be a public health issue because what hurts them might end up hurting their patients.

Because of MedRAP's efficient design, maximum benefits for residency programs can be achieved with a judicious commitment of time and resources. MedRAP effectively addresses both the ACGME competencies and residents' well-being with an efficient use of resources.

I have written this book with the hope that by describing the MedRAP method, other institutions will be encouraged to develop similar training programs to improve professional development and the overall work environment, in order to enhance the well-being of their residents, other health care professionals and, ultimately, patients.

If my experience can help improve the well-being of health care professionals, perhaps it can serve as a small ripple effect in the medical community that becomes a positive force for change, since what helps the physician also helps the patient.

Iris C. Mushin, M.Ed., MBA

ACKNOWLEDGEMENTS

To the multiple generations of MedRAP senior resident group leaders who worked tirelessly and altruistically to help improve the training environment, the professional development of their subordinates, hospital efficiency, and patient care, I owe my deepest thanks.

I am deeply indebted to Dr. Antonio M. Gotto, Chair of Internal Medicine when I launched MedRAP, for allowing this program to come to fruition at Baylor College of Medicine and initially supporting it financially. I am also grateful to the following Baylor College of Medicine Faculty who assisted me with this program. I am thankful that Dr. Edward C. Lynch understood the need for the program and actively assisted me in its launch. Dr. Stephen B. Greenberg supported the program for many years as the Chair of Internal Medicine at Ben Taub, and later as the Chair of the Internal Medicine Department and Dean of Graduate Medical Education at Baylor College of Medicine. I would like to acknowledge the assistance and support of the late Dr. Ralph D. Feigin, Physician–in–Chief at Texas Children's Hospital, as well as President and CEO of Baylor College of Medicine. I greatly appreciate Dr. Amir Halevy for his strong advocacy and sustained support for MedRAP while he served as the Internal Medicine Residency Program Director. He courageously stood up for his principles in his mission to improve the house staff training experience, and was a strong supporter of MedRAP. He also provided me with valuable insight and critique during the writing of this book. Another Internal Medicine Program Director, Dr. Richard J. Hamill, was very helpful throughout the years I worked with him. Dr. William A. Myerson, the Director of the Department of Medicine's Behavioral Medicine Programs, served on the initial MedRAP advisory committee. He brought a unique perspective and provided valuable guidance and opportunities that helped shape the program. I also appreciate the insight he offered while I was writing this book.

MedRAP was conceived while I was an MBA student and developed under the supervision of Dr. Michael T. Matteson, Chair of the Department of Organizational Behavior and Management at the University of Houston Bauer College of Business. I am grateful for his guidance and everything he taught me about organizations. Ellen Gittess was instrumental in providing me with professional advice throughout the years, and I am grateful for her wisdom, advice and commitment. I would like to thank Sasha Alexander for her sincere commitment to MedRAP and for her unwavering belief in the program goals and impact. I deeply appreciate the many ways she supported me, participating in the MedRAP sessions and contributing to the facilitator manual editing. Joy Haley helped me create the book I envisioned with her thoughtful editorial comments. I am grateful for her support, commitment to the project, and for her friendship. I could not have written this book without the help, dedication and commitment of my long-time administrative assistant, Debbie Arcy, who served in multiple roles with great competence and professionalism. My wonderful family understood how important it was for me to write this book so that MedRAP would live on and continue to help future generations. They offered limitless support, endless patience and unconditional love.

SECTION 1

FOUNDATIONAL CONCEPTS AND DESIGN

This section provides a detailed description of a Medical Residents' Assistance Program (MedRAP) designed to enhance the well-being and professional development of medical trainees. The program utilizes concepts and principles from various disciplines, including organizational, psychological, and educational theory, to create an integrated and comprehensive program. The chapters in this section discuss the need for changes in post-graduate medical training and the advantages of MedRAP's specific approach.

CHAPTER 1:

HEALING HEALTH CARE THROUGH IMPROVED MEDICAL TRAINING

A robust health care system requires healthy physicians. This statement may seem self-evident; however, traditional efforts to improve health care systems have focused on decreasing costs and improving access. It is only recently that more attention is being paid to physicians' well-being and wellness; studies have demonstrated that without physicians who feel engaged, valued, and fairly treated, a health care delivery system cannot function optimally.[1,2]

In recent years, the health care practice environment has changed significantly, creating additional substantial stressors for physicians and leading to declining physician satisfaction and well-being. These stressors include lack of resources, erosion of professional autonomy and loss of control, changes in the insurance industry and decline in compensation, time-constrained patient care, and increased clerical burden.[3-6] As a result, the prevalence of stress and burnout among physicians is higher than in any other comparable professional group and twice the rate of the general population of the United States.[7] National studies report that about half of the physicians in the U.S. are experiencing professional burnout.[8]

The work that physicians perform is different from the daily activities of the average businessperson. Physicians wrestle daily with life-and-death issues and experience the fear, pain, and grief of patients and their families. They carry an emotional burden that sets their work apart from that of other professionals. Unwell physicians are at an increased risk for substance abuse, relationship problems, depression, and even death. Physicians also experience higher rates of emotional exhaustion and depression, as well as substance abuse, troubled marriages, and divorce.[9-14]

According to the American Foundation for Suicide Prevention, physicians are twice as likely to commit suicide as non-physicians, with 300 to 400 doctors committing suicide every year[15]—more than double the rate in the general population and the equivalent of two to three graduating medical school classes.

This phenomenon cuts across all ages, stages, and career paths—from trainees to senior practitioners—and these challenges are not unique to physicians. Nurses and other clinicians experience similar effects on performance, health, and well-being.

It is critical to keep in mind that unwell physicians affect more than just themselves. Studies indicate that unwellness in medical staff can reduce workplace productivity and efficiency. For example, a reduction in physician well-being can increase the practice of defensive medicine, which is reflected in unnecessary tests or procedures. There is a correlation between physician stress and burnout and negative effects on clinical practice, including increased medical errors, suboptimal care, unprofessional behavior, decreased patient satisfaction, and increased malpractice litigation.[16-18] Stressed and burned-out physicians can also negatively impact colleagues who rely on them, potentially jeopardizing the function of their health care team.

Another potentially long-term consequence of burnout has recently emerged: a shortage of physicians has been projected by the U.S. Department of Health and Human Services by 2025. Professional burnout is one factor that may have been underestimated in causing this shortage.[19] The plan is to address this shortage by recruiting international medical graduates. However, immigrant doctors may experience burnout due to cultural adjustments and the unique stressors and strains they are likely to face, above and beyond those that they share with their U.S. trained colleagues.

Stress is often expected to be intense when working in the health care industry and taking care of patients. Health professionals encounter unique stressors that begin in medical school and continue throughout their career.[20] However, medical institutions often contribute to this stress by having an organizational culture where leadership is not supportive and negative policies are implemented. These can include: (1) emphasizing hierarchy while discounting the importance of teams and collaboration, which often hinders communication, trust, and innovation; (2) an inefficient environment where there is difficulty in providing timely, optimal care to patients.[17,21]

Given the magnitude of potential safety issues and organization-wide financial impacts, the toll of physician unwellness, stress, and burnout has far more serious consequences than in other professions.[8,22] The high burnout rate reported in U.S. physicians highlights a serious problem in the health care delivery system; in order to improve population health and patients' experiences and reduce the cost of care, it is essential to improve the well-being and work-life of physicians and other health care professionals.[3]

A NOTE ON WELL-BEING AND WELLNESS

Wellness and well-being are general terms which are increasingly mentioned and sometimes used interchangeably in medical literature. For the purpose of this book, well-being and wellness are defined as follows:

Physician **well-being** is a broad term which describes the physician's sense of engagement, purpose, resilience, satisfaction, high level of morale, and success in various aspects of personal and professional life.

Physician **wellness** describes the state of being in good physical and mental health.

"If a physician's personal well-being is measured on a continuum, then wellness and burnout may represent opposing poles of the scale".[23]

THE IMPACT OF GRADUATE MEDICAL EDUCATION (GME)

Unfortunately, for medical professionals, the seeds of unwellness are often planted in the formative years of medical school and residency.[24] Perhaps this is because transitions in medical education are reported to be an especially strained period when many new stressors are encountered. The first year of residency (internship), when medical students transition into residency, can be particularly difficult. Many residents are required to move to a new place, are often heavily in debt as a result of their medical education, are required to work long hours, and are mistreated at times by senior staff.[15,25,26] Rates of depression and burnout in the first year of residency are reported to increase from 4% to 55%.[13,24,27-32]

PGY-1 (post-graduate, year one) residents also have to adapt to new clinical responsibilities in unfamiliar and challenging working environments, which is reported to lead to stress and burnout, mental health problems, and poor patient care. In fact, studies show that medical residents are particularly vulnerable to stress, depression, and burnout, with overall prevalence ranging from 25% to as high as 75%, depending on the specialty.[33]

Non-supportive training and working environments have been widely acknowledged as major contributors to burnout, stress, and unprofessional conduct. The surprisingly high prevalence of harassment and discrimination during medical training has not declined over time.[34] The frequency of mistreatment in the training environment has negative implications for professionalism and makes it difficult to instill virtuous behavior. Harassment and discrimination has a profound negative impact on residents' health and well-being. As recently as 2014, a study identified that the prevalence of mistreatment during medical training continues to be a persistent problem. It was reported that 59.4% of medical trainees had experienced harassment or discrimination during their training.[34,35]

Numerous studies have established that highly stressed, burned-out physicians are also more likely to be dissatisfied and unprofessional, and that this phenomenon is prevalent. Unfortunately, evidence suggests that many post-graduate medical education programs fail to assist in the acquisition and development of the qualities that contribute to professionalism. [36-38] Declining professionalism and cynicism on the part of physician mentors in the post-graduate medical education setting is a significant negative influence on trainees.[39]

Although the transformation of an individual into a skilled medical professional is a gradual and complex social process that occurs throughout all phases of medical education, residency is reported to be the time when the work habits of physicians are established. The time spent in post-graduate training—and the experiences residents encounter during these formative years—have a lasting effect on the type of doctors they will become, as well as how readily they will be able to cope with environments that pose significant threats to their well-being and professionalism.[33,40-43]

In order to function effectively, succeed in their new work and training environment, reduce their stress, and maintain a high level of morale, residents require a set of core skills that are often not taught in the formal curriculum. For example, residents often lack adequate organizational, interpersonal, and leadership skills.[44] Some schools offer a "Transition to Internship"[25] course in the fourth year of medical school. However, residents report that assistance and guidance during the first year of residency (when they actually assume direct responsibilities for patient care and will encounter new challenges) would be less esoteric, more relevant, and would accelerate their learning curve more effectively.[43]

THE NEGATIVE IMPLICATIONS OF BURNOUT AMONG HEALTH CARE PROFESSIONALS

BURNOUT AND DEPRESSION AMONG PHYSICIANS

Burnout and stress impact commitment and dedication among health care professionals, as well as cause erosion in professionalism, reduction in quality of care, and increased medical errors. Studies suggest that:

- Professional burnout is experienced by at least half of U.S. physicians[1,18]
- The prevalence of burnout among U.S. physicians is higher than among their peers in the general population[45]
- Burnout among U.S. physicians is getting worse[4]
- Physicians' work-related stress negatively impacts patient outcome[2]
- More than 50% of physicians believe that tiredness, exhaustion, or sleep deprivation negatively affect patient care[38]
- Recruitment and retention rates plummet as stress and burnout increases[4]
- Physicians who are highly dissatisfied with their work have increased probability of changing jobs within medicine or leaving medicine entirely[4]
- Unhappy physicians are more likely to provide suboptimal care, such as prescribing inappropriate medications, which can lead to costly complications[37]
- As stress increases, turnover rates rise and contribute to the increasing costs associated with recruitment and retention of physicians; excessive job stress, burnout, and dissatisfaction are closely related to job and career turnover[4]
- The total cost of replacing one family physician approaches $250,000[2]
- Physicians are twice as likely to commit suicide as non-physicians[26]
- An average of 300-400 doctors commit suicide every year[46]
- Stress and burnout experienced by physicians impedes recruitment of the best and the brightest individuals into medicine and into some medical specialties[4]
- The burnout rate for medical faculty has been reported to range between 20 and 49%[47]

BURNOUT AND DEPRESSION IN MEDICAL TRAINING

- Medical training involves numerous risk factors for mental illness, such as role transition, decreased sleep, relocation resulting in fewer available support systems, and feelings of isolation[15]
- Distress and burnout peak during medical training[45]
- Rates of burnout in the first year of residency are reported to increase from 4% to 55%[13]
- About one third of medical residents report depressive symptoms in the first year of residency training[38]
- Medical trainees have higher rates of depression than other graduate students in the general public[48]
- Burnt-out residents have been identified as being significantly more likely to provide suboptimal patient care or commit medical errors[2]
- Despite the fact that medical trainees are at high risk for depression and suicidal thoughts, training programs have not been able to provide treatment for these residents and fellows in a systematic way[15]

THE TIME FOR CHANGE IS NOW

Given the significant impact on public health, the toll of professional burnout has far more profound consequences than in other professions. What hurts the physician ultimately hurts the patient, and today's physicians are hurting. This epidemic of burnout among doctors, and its negative impact on health care, is increasingly seen as an issue of public health. Indeed, the general public has begun to recognize this escalating problem, as evidenced by mainstream media reports on this issue, including "Taking Care of the Physician" published in the *NY-Times* (2017); "Why Do Doctors Commit Suicide?" published in the *NY-Times* (2014); "Life/Support: Inside the Movement to Save the Mental Health of Today's Doctors," published by *Time* magazine (September 1, 2015); and "Doctors Are Human Too," published by the *NY-Times* (International edition, April 21, 2017).

REPORTED BURNOUT RATES BY SPECIALTY[24]

- Dermatology 50%
- Family Medicine 27%
- General Surgery 40%
- Internal Medicine 63%
- Neurology 63%
- Obstetrics/Gynecology 75%
- Ophthalmology 60%
- Pediatrics 55-60%
- Psychiatry 40%

To respond to the problem, the National Academy of Medicine (NAM) established the ***Action Collaborative on Clinician Well-Being and Resilience*** in 2016 to build a collaborative platform for supporting and improving clinician well-being and resilience across multiple organizations. This important initiative can help ensure the well-being of all health care professionals, thereby impacting the whole system.[2,47,49] It can also help serve as a measure of the health care industry's overall quality.

The cost of stress in the health care industry is immense.[2,50,51] Solutions to this problem remain limited, but there is growing understanding of the importance of both promoting physician well-being and improving the organizational culture within medical institutions.[2] Stress-reduction techniques can assist individuals; however, a systems approach is required to effectively address a problem generated by the organizational culture. A systems-based approach recognizes that stress and depression leading to burnout, suicide, or other unhealthy behaviors represent a culmination of multiple factors that impact well-being.

Institutional commitment to physician well-being programs can greatly assist in addressing the current crisis of physician burnout and dissatisfaction. Combining institutional approaches—which include reshaping organizational cultures, working environments, and promoting efforts to improve individual physicians' well-being—seems to present the best intervention. There is also a substantial business argument to be made in favor of creating a workplace that fosters satisfaction among health care staff, since it leads to a significant competitive advantage. Investing in physician well-being helps improve patient satisfaction, which impacts cost of care and reimbursement.[1,47,52,53]

Medical institutions have begun to realize there is a need to find practical, cost-effective ways to help their practicing health care professionals cope with the challenges of modern medical practice[1] so they can:

- Provide high quality of care
- Contribute to patient satisfaction
- Function effectively and efficiently

More needs to be done by health care leadership to understand and address these important problems. Health care institutions will benefit from utilizing organizational interventions to foster a positive organizational culture and empower health care professionals and medical trainees to report mistreatment or systematic problems without fear of retribution. Such an approach will also contribute to enhancing well-being, professional development, and professionalism—something lectures and ethics seminars alone cannot do.

It is possible for medical education programs and health care institutions to integrate well-being, wellness, and resiliency activities into all aspects of education and training in the organization. Effective interventions can be relatively inexpensive and can have a large return on investment.[53,54] Creating systems to support medical trainees and health care professionals can also promote the development of future leaders who can help cultivate and foster positive working environments where health care professionals can thrive.[51]

Optimal data on ways to improve well-being and reduce stress and burnout requires further research and will take time. However, providers' well-being, stress, and burnout need to be addressed *now*. Medical institutions can utilize effective models that have been successfully implemented, rather than waiting for further study results. Too much is at stake.

CHAPTER 2:
HOW MEDRAP CAN HELP MEDICAL INSTITUTIONS

MedRAP is an effective, comprehensive and integrated program designed to advance the professional and personal growth of young medical clinicians, improve their well-being and work environment, and help reduce stress and burnout. The program positively impacted the working and training environment of medical residents in Baylor College of Medicine's (BCM) Department of Internal Medicine for more than two decades by applying organizational, psychological, and educational insight to help residents meet the challenges they commonly encountered in their training.

Implementation of MedRAP at BCM confirmed that investing in physician well-being fosters physicians who take better care of their patients, who in turn will be more satisfied with their care. These investments benefit physicians, their patients, and the health care industry as a whole.

INSTITUTIONAL BENEFITS

MedRAP would not have existed successfully for so many years had it not met unsolved needs for both institutional management and individual residents. Taking care of the provider's team is a critical part of achieving the organization's goals and offers a return on investment through greater functional efficiency and increased patient satisfaction and reimbursement.[1]

MedRAP provides a forum for early detection of organizational problems and systemic issues, as well as a safety net to

APPLICABILITY OF THIS BOOK

The lessons and skills developed in this book are cross-applicable to many realms in medicine. While MedRAP was originally designed to help physician trainees, the program can be tailored to the needs of practicing medical professionals, non-physician trainees and providers, and administration.

catch otherwise quality physicians in danger of succumbing to burnout or mal-adaptive behaviors. The program's ability to identify early adjustment problems faced by individuals can help preserve a hospital's substantial investment in recruitment, training and retention of new physicians.

From an operations standpoint, the Quality Improvement (QI) component creates an opportunity for greater efficiencies, potentially contributing to cost savings. QI involves the entire health care team in improving collaboration, bringing positive organizational change, and enabling early identification of organizational problems that residents experience related to clinical care and hospital efficiency.

Systematic errors are identified through specifically designed questionnaires tailored to each affiliated hospital. Potential solutions are then formulated and presented to the program director, administration, and the management of the health care team in each affiliated hospital. This process facilitates collaboration between the residents, residency program directors, faculty, and health care team members, and can break down many of the invisible barriers often experienced by these groups.

From an accreditation standpoint, MedRAP addresses competencies required by the Accreditation Council for Graduate Medical Education (ACGME). In 1999, the ACGME and American Board of Medical Specialties (ABMS) established core competencies, requiring residency and fellowship programs to ensure that medical trainees master a wide range of professional competencies and specific milestones assigned to each.

MedRAP was developed in 1988, more than a decade before the ACGME Outcome Project established the competency-based education. At that time, the program had already identified that communication skills, organizational skills, leadership skills, and management skills are essential components of professional maturation. The program recognized that these skills were ideally developed during residency and were as important to the quality of medical care as the acquisition of academic skills. MedRAP addresses several ACGME requirements, including milestones within:

- Interpersonal and communication skills
- Professionalism
- Systems-based practice
- Practice-based learning and improvement
- Patient care

MedRAP also responds to additional ACGME requirements. For example, ACGME requires that the hospital provide supportive training environments, free from discrimination or harassment. Residency programs should establish an organizational system for residents to communicate and exchange information; foster an educational environment in which residents can resolve issues confidentially; and provide individual assistance in responding to situational, personal, and professional stress.

The table highlights some of the key skills taught to residents, along with their associated ROI and ACGME competencies. Each section is color coded to correspond to the related chapters.

SUMMARY OF KEY INSTITUTIONAL BENEFITS

▶ Early identification of organizational problems

▶ Early identification of individual adjustment problems

▶ Facilitation of collaboration among the entire health care team

▶ Quality Improvement (QI) in the affiliated hospitals

▶ Assistance with recruitment and retention of house staff

SKILLS AND COMPETENCIES	RETURN ON INVESTMENT (ROI)	ACGME COMPETENCIES AND MILESTONES ADDRESSED*
Organizational Skills	• Helps to reduce the impact of cohort turnover • Accelerates transitions during academic changeovers • Helps improve residents' efficiency	• Practice-Based Learning and Improvement • Patient Care • Interpersonal and Communications Skills
Communication Skills	• Improves communication and collaboration with patients, their families, and the health care team • Contributes to patient satisfaction, which is linked to cost of care and reimbursement • Contributes to improved quality of code status discussion • Promotes effective management of negative feelings towards patients and families that can interfere in care • Assists with risk management	• Interpersonal and Communications Skills • Professionalism
Quality Improvement / Management Skills	• Facilitates early identification of problems • Improves hospital efficiency • Improves collaboration with health care team • Improves efficiency of patient care • Increases physicians' participation in improving health care delivery	• Systems-Based Practice • Practice-Based Learning and Improvement
Leadership Skills	• Increases efficient functioning of team leaders • Improves educational experience of residents • Improves patient care by minimizing impact of cohort changeovers	• Professionalism • Interpersonal and Communications Skills
Annual Evaluation and Planning	• Ensures ongoing evolution of program, to continue providing an effective response to participants' and management's needs	

*See Present Requirements Competencies table at the end of every topic chapter for specific milestones addressed.

MEDRAP TIME AND RESOURCE COMMITMENTS

Now more than ever, with the rising cost of health care, hospital leadership, administrators, and care team managers are under increasing pressure to allocate resources efficiently and optimize patient care with limited resources.[2]

MedRAP's efficient design provides substantial benefits for the residency program and affiliated hospitals, which can be achieved with a reasonable commitment of time, taking into consideration the extensive demands of residency. The time and resource commitments are negligible when considering the return on investment MedRAP provides.

Senior resident group leaders (GLs) commit two hours monthly to GL meetings, and two hours monthly to the PGY-1 meetings. In return, GLs develop and build their own leadership skills while also earning management recognition for their contribution to the residency program. PGY-1 residents attend a monthly two-hour meeting.

TIME COMMITMENT:

- PGY-1 residents: 2 hours each month
- GLs: PGY-2 and PGY-3 residents spend 4 hours each month (GLs meeting and PGY-1 session)
- During February and March, selected GLs who participate in preparing and presenting QI presentations spend additional 4-6 hours
- Facilitator: conducts and facilitates all the GL and PGY-1 sessions; tailors the program to the needs of the PGY-1 residents through a needs analysis, with the assistance of the GLs
  - ◉ Time commitment of facilitator depends upon the size and needs of the residency program
  - ◉ The initial year of implementation requires more time to tailor the materials to the individual program needs
  - ◉ In subsequent years, and on an ongoing basis, facilitators can assume planning and individual consulting time of 2 hours per GL session and 1 hour per PGY-1 session, in addition to facilitating all the sessions

RESIDENCY PROGRAM RESOURCE COMMITMENT:

- Administrative assistance for:
  - ◉ Creating demographically balanced PGY-1 groups
  - ◉ Booking conference rooms
  - ◉ Ordering lunches
  - ◉ Email and phone reminders about meetings and rescheduling meetings if needed
  - ◉ Phone reminders by the residency program personnel help ensure that PGY-1 residents can be relieved from their clinical responsibilities and allowed to attend or reschedule when they are on call or have an emergency
  - ◉ Scheduling and preparing QI presentations
  - ◉ Parking if needed
  - ◉ Audiovisual equipment if needed
- The facilitator's salary optimally is provided by the medical school or the residency training program
- When the mixed faculty model is utilized (described in Chapter 4), other forms of compensation can also be developed, such as educational credit tied to promotion or relief from some clinical responsibilities

RESIDENT BENEFITS

One of the most notable advantages to the MedRAP program is that it creates a mutually-beneficial situation for institutions and physicians. The benefits of improved well-being and stress reduction of health care professionals mirror themselves in corresponding institutional benefits of operational efficiencies and improved patient care.

Physicians need to see that their health care organization values the well-being of its staff, and endeavors to cultivate an efficient and positive work environment. Implementing programs such as MedRAP demonstrates this commitment. MedRAP accelerates residents' transition from medical school to residency, providing them with tools to function more effectively in the hospital work environment, which contributes to their well-being.

Because the MedRAP program begins with a needs analysis followed by the development of curriculum specific to the identified stressors, it is uniquely proactive in its approach. Strategies and tools are provided to handle challenges residents are likely to experience in their specific rotations, hospitals, and specialties. The curriculum includes discussion and activities meant to teach residents how to constructively address common stressors.

The ongoing confidential feedback collection, as well as the QI component, allows residents to provide suggestions on how to remove or alleviate these stressors and bring constructive change to the hospital work environment. Empowering the house staff to make a difference contributes to resident well-being, reduces burnout, increases professionalism, and helps improve care.[3] Without the safe environment, residents may observe and encounter inefficiencies in patient care, yet not feel comfortable reporting or addressing them. Physician reluctance to relay inefficiencies causes additional frustration among house staff who lack training in the organizational techniques imperative to produce change.

MedRAP also provides an individual assistance component for those residents experiencing personal and professional adjustment issues with their transition to residency.

SUMMARY OF KEY RESIDENT BENEFITS

▸ Accelerates residents' transition from medical school to residency, and subsequently into practice

▸ Provides residents with skills that contribute to their professional development

▸ Anticipates and identifies stressors residents are likely to experience

▸ Utilizes strategies to alleviate stress

▸ Facilitates a positive and effective training environment

▸ Empowers residents to improve their work environment

▸ Provides individual assistance, as needed

MEDRAP'S UNIQUE ADVANTAGE

MedRAP is not alone, but it is unique. The health care industry has increasingly recognized the institutional and individual benefits of producing well physicians. All GME programs are now required to develop core competencies and evaluate trainees' progress in meeting the milestones mandated by the ACGME. Various GME programs have been developed to improve the professional development of medical trainees.[4-10] Several programs improve well-being and reduce stress and burnout,[11-16] foster professionalism,[12,17-20] and train in health care improvement methods.[21-27] However, programs to reduce stress and burnout before it results in impairment are not common, and data on these programs is scarce.[11] In addition, no other program describes an intervention that is as comprehensive, integrated, and all-inclusive as MedRAP.

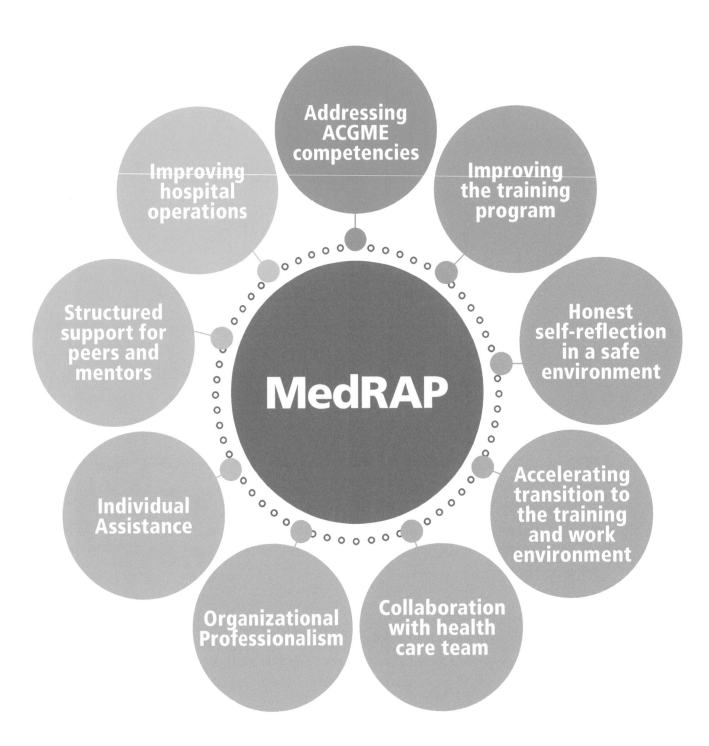

**MedRAP is a uniquely comprehensive program
that promotes professional development
and well-being in medical residents.**

CHAPTER 3:

THE MEDRAP APPROACH: ADDRESSING REAL VS. ASSUMED NEEDS

As already discussed, to ensure the well-being of physicians and other health care professionals, it is imperative for medical institutions to cultivate a positive organizational environment that promotes professional development and well-being, associated with decreased levels of stress and burnout. However, rather than treating the symptoms after they occur, it is more effective and efficient to identify what contributes to health care professionals' stress and burnout, and then develop preventative measures in order to improve their well-being. Preventative programs can also facilitate a culture change, when needed, in graduate medical education.[1-3]

MedRAP was developed at BCM based on these concepts, and through the 25 years of its implementation, it was preventative in nature. The program continuously evolved based on the specific needs of the participants and the organization. MedRAP's success demonstrated that it is possible to facilitate an effective transition from medical school to residency by anticipating and alleviating many of the difficulties previously experienced by residents. Participants reported that receiving assistance with their transition during residency, when they were facing significantly different challenges, was actually more effective than their preparation courses in medical school.

In order to formulate an effective program that addressed real rather than assumed needs, a thorough needs analysis was conducted to identify the actual stressors encountered by residents. Discussion on how to run a needs assessment is included in Chapter 5.

During the needs assessment, seven core resident stressors were identified, many of which are common among residency programs. Each of these stressors was then addressed in the core curriculum and structure. The seven identified stressors and MedRAP's response to them are discussed in the following pages.

STRESSOR #1:

Morale was low, and residents felt burned out; these feelings impacted the way they related to their patients.

Burnout can impact the safety of a large number of patients treated in academic hospitals. The majority of them will be treated at some point by a resident. A broadly applicable description defines "burnout" as a state of mental and physical exhaustion related to work or caregiving activities. An expanded definition also characterizes the symptoms of burnout as emotional exhaustion (emotional overextension and fatigue), depersonalization (negative, callous, detached responses to others), and a reduced perception of personal accomplishment (feelings of incompetence and poor achievement in one's work).[4]

Duty-hours reform has been the major focus of addressing resident burnout.[5] In 2003, the ACGME implemented work-hour limitations. The work week was cut down to 80 hours. Preliminary studies indicated that work-hour limitations had improved some aspects of residents' quality of life. However, data suggests that burnout rates did not decrease in concert with the reduction in work hours.[2] Studies reported that the prevalence of burnout in residents still exceeded 40%, even after residency programs implemented the ACGME-mandated work-hour limitations.[6,7] Residents suffering from stress and burnout can pose as much risk to patients as exhausted residents, regardless of their fatigue level, due to increased potential for medical mistakes.[8]

Negative training environments have also been widely acknowledged as major contributors to stress, burnout, and unprofessional conduct.[9] The frequency of this complaint suggests that the origin of the problem lies in the system rather than with the individuals.

MedRAP facilitates a more effective transition for residents by identifying problems they are likely to encounter at the beginning of the year, and throughout the year at the beginning of new rotations. They are provided with tools and strategies—developed with the assistance of their group leaders—to help them handle these anticipated problems more effectively, thus reducing their stress and enhancing the effectiveness of patient care.

The program is designed to improve residents' well-being, associated with reduced burnout, increased professionalism, and improved patient care and satisfaction, by:[10,11]

- Establishing a supportive and safe environment to encourage honest feedback
- Providing structured mentor and peer support
- Promoting candid self-reflection

- Facilitating and accelerating effective transitions
- Improving their efficiency and effectiveness as physicians
- Empowering them to solve organizational problems and increasing their sense of control over their work and training environment

Some of the most valuable training an employee receives is the informal instruction that occurs through interactions with co-workers. Effective professional development programs integrate this informal learning with the formal training. However, most residency programs have not yet emphasized this integration, and the collective wisdom of past generations is often not effectively communicated to PGY-1 residents. They are left to "reinvent the wheel"—not always with the best results. As a consequence, a great deal of unnecessary stress is introduced into the training process.[12]

STRESSOR #2:

Residents were often ill-equipped to deal with the clinical and non-clinical responsibilities encountered during the first year of training, such as:

1) Managing time effectively

2) Coping with new and varied responsibilities

3) Navigating the different hospital systems

4) Dealing with difficult interactions with patients, their families, senior staff, and paraprofessional personnel

At times, new house staff can acquire maladaptive coping strategies as a result of informal training and the hidden curriculum. For example, senior residents may embody norms and values that residents begin to reflect—even if these norms and values are contrary to the formal curriculum. Since the MedRAP approach formalizes the random training that residents encounter in hospitals and health systems, and anticipates typical problems and best practices to handle them ahead of time, the program helps ensure that imparted strategies in the informal training are adaptive rather than maladaptive. It is important to address both the informal and hidden curriculum of health care academic organizations, which do not always support the formal professional development curriculum.

The program facilitator works directly with senior residents to develop a more consistent transfer of the collective wisdom regarding how to function effectively in a clinical environment. The program also provides structured coaching, feedback, mentorship, leadership training, and team-building for participants. This system helps the organization recognize professional issues that might otherwise go unaddressed.

FORMAL CURRICULUM: The official standard educational platform for residents in each teaching institute.

INFORMAL CURRICULUM: Teaching and learning that randomly occurs outside of the formal curriculum in a variety of settings and ward rotations in residency; can include tips and tools on how to be organizationally efficient, how to respond to communication challenges, and how to succeed with the information and practices imparted; can be consistent or inconsistent with the formal curriculum.

HIDDEN CURRICULUM: Unintended lessons that are learned during residency that may be contrary to the formal curriculum. The hidden curriculum reflects the organizational culture of the residency program and influences the norms and values that residents assimilate.[13]

The curriculum addresses problems residents are likely to encounter in several areas, providing best practices, tools, and strategies to handle these challenges.

- Organizational skills
  - Time management
  - Priority-setting
  - Tips on navigating the system
- Communication skills
  - With patients
  - With patients' family members
  - With fellow health care team members
- Leadership skills
  - Providing constructive feedback
  - Team-building methods
  - Effective teaching
- Management skills
  - Identifying systemic errors
  - Developing skills to solve organizational/systemic problems encountered
  - Collaborating with the health care team to improve care

Traditionally, physician mentors have served as role models for residents. However, with the growing demands of patient care, increased size of training programs, busy public hospitals, and ACGME working-hours require-ments, this type of relationship is becoming increasingly difficult and more problematic. Insufficient pro-fessional mentorship can compromise residents' ability to provide optimal and safe patient care, decreasing their access to vital information and limiting their potential capacity to instruct others. Deficient mentorship is also reflected in the failure of some senior residents to maintain professionalism when assuming the role of mentor and educator.[14]

STRESSOR #3:

The residents reported that their mentorship experiences, which could significantly impact their performance, were inconsistent, varying from month to month depending on the abilities and skills of their senior resident team leaders.

Health care professional trainees actively learn from their seniors in the hospital work environment, and this learning represents a major component in their ability to function effectively as physicians. To help ensure that mentorship relationships are supportive rather than stressful and punitive, organizations can provide preparation and support for future mentors.[12,15]

MedRAP structures the mentorship experience by utilizing a specially-designed technique to select and train senior residents as group leaders (GLs) for small groups of PGY-1 residents. The group leaders assist the PGY-1 residents in learning how to professionally handle the problems they are likely to encounter. Role models are a powerful way for young doctors to learn respect, empathy, and other professional behaviors, and effective mentorship is associated with greater staff satisfaction and well-being. The involvement of senior residents in the program provides residents with an additional opportunity to further develop such relationships. Research has shown that it is important to cultivate peer and mentor relationships through which organizational values can be role-modeled and supported.[16]

When mechanisms for honest feedback are absent, it prevents early identi-fication of and solutions to problems that residents experience in their training and work environment in the hospital wards. This can lead to frustration, stress, and burnout among the resi-dents. PGY-1 residents are often not comfortable communicating feedback about their training and work expe-riences to their superiors because they don't want to be perceived as complainers or trouble-makers. Even if they do provide feedback,

STRESSOR # 4:

Residents were concerned about retribution from senior residents, faculty nurses, or other health care team members when providing feedback related to both their training and work experiences. As a result, important information that could impact patient care was not being communicated.

this information is often not communicated to the program management. It is important to accelerate the flow of information all the way from the residents to the management of the residency training program. Doing so on an ongoing basis can help improve the educational experience of residents, as well as lead to better patient care.

MedRAP includes a structured time for residents to provide confidential feedback within each session. Since the program is operationally independent from the formal residency program, it contributes to a safe environment that facilitates early detection and solutions to problems—both on the personal and organizational levels—without fear of repercussions. The information is communicated monthly to chief residents or the program management, which addresses the problems the residents experience in their training and work environment. Time is also allocated at the end of each session for individual residents to address personal or professional adjustment issues.

STRESSOR #5:

The residents were frustrated with the inefficiency and ineffectiveness of the hospital work environment in some of the affiliated hospital systems.

Physicians' daily work requires the intellect to evaluate and develop solutions to complex problems in patient care.[17] They are trained to pay attention to details, think critically, and base their decisions on evidence. This combination of skills can also be utilized in improving organizational efficiency and effectiveness and can lead to a participatory management approach.

In addition to collecting ongoing feedback in a safe environment, MedRAP includes a QI component. This component is an organizational approach designed by MedRAP to improve residents' management and systems-based practice skills and involve them, annually, in:

(1) identifying and solving organizational problems present in the hospital work environment,
(2) accelerating the flow of information to hospital administration, and
(3) improving collaboration with colleagues and the health care team.

STRESSOR #6:

Residents felt isolated because they did not have enough opportunities to interact with peers, share experiences, or self-reflect on difficult emotional issues they were encountering.

Being involved in improving the work environment has been demonstrated in industry to lead to improved morale and a sense of empowerment, which is associated with burnout reduction.[18-20]

Difficult situations encountered during residents' training can lead to a variety of negative emotional consequences, including a sense of isolation, depression, and anxiety. It is important that they do not feel alone under these circumstances.[21]

Residents need to be able to share their feelings, vulnerabilities, and difficulties in challenging situations, such as when they pronounce death, when they make a medical mistake, or when they lose a patient under their care. A training culture that encourages them to be honest and acknowledge their vulnerabilities can help them be more responsive to patients, more likely to ask for help with difficult cases, and more adept at working effectively on a team. Creating a supportive community and providing peer support in a safe environment has been reported to promote emotional growth and professional development of postgraduate medical trainees. This type of support can make them better doctors.[22,23]

MedRAP provides this safe environment where residents can share experiences, self-reflect, and learn from peers and mentors how to deal with difficulties they encounter. The highly-structured nature of the sessions is helpful because it allows a variety of typically-encountered problems to be considered, rather than concentrating for a long period on a few issues. The structure of the sessions also prevents the meetings from turning into gripe sessions, and maintains the problem-solving orientation.

For many physicians, seeking help carries a discouraging stigma. Studies report that more than 80% of general practitioners and hospital doctors work through illnesses. Results from interviews with doctors show that professional and organizational barriers reinforce one another and could contribute to a prevailing

> ## STRESSOR #7:
>
> The residents felt there was a need for a place where they could receive confidential assistance to deal with personal or professional adjustment issues.

reluctance to take sick leave or discuss personal health concerns with colleagues.[24] Doctors may feel uncomfortable assuming the role of patient for fear that others will interpret their need for help as an indicator of their inability to cope with professional challenges.[25,26]

Physicians may also be deterred from seeking help for physical or mental health issues, as well as substance abuse problems, out of fear that licensing boards will discriminate against them—even in instances where the diagnosis has no effect on their professional performance or when effective treatment has already been received.[27,28] Many medical licensing applications include questions regarding physical health, mental health, and substance use of applicants.[29] Some licensing boards undertake investigations if physicians seek treatment, which can lead to sanctions irrespective of whether there is any evidence of impaired functioning.[30]

Physicians can have difficulty exhibiting professional behaviors when they must personally deal with the serious personal or work-related adjustment issues that impact their lives. These issues can affect patient care. MedRAP has a built-in mechanism for individual assistance, which helps physicians deal confidentially with personal and professional adjustment issues on an ongoing basis within the health care training institution or externally, if needed.

SECTION 2

PROGRAM STRUCTURE AND IMPLEMENTATION

The following chapters provide a detailed description of MedRAP's overall design and the key steps to implementation.

CHAPTER 4:

PROGRAM OVERVIEW

MEDRAP MISSION STATEMENT

MedRAP is a comprehensive program designed to advance the professional and personal growth of young medical clinicians, improve their well-being and work environment, and reduce stress and burnout. The program focuses on developing competencies such as professionalism, communication and interpersonal skills, and systems-based practice skills. The Quality Improvement (QI) component of the program is designed to involve the entire health care team in improving collaboration and bringing positive organizational change to the hospital work environment.

MedRAP follows a 12-month schedule addressing the evolving needs of residents. This chapter will explain the flow of the program curriculum, the structure of MedRAP sessions for group leaders and PGY-1 residents, and MedRAP facilitators' tips on designing effective sessions.

MONTHS 1 - 2
Orientation and Organizational Skills

The MedRAP program implementation officially starts for PGY-1 residents in June. Facilitators meet with the selected GLs to orient them to MedRAP's goals, provide group leadership training, and prepare material for the departmental orientation. (GL selection process is explained in Chapter 5.)

At the end of the Department of Medicine orientation, previously selected MedRAP GLs meet with the PGY-1 residents in their pre-assigned small groups for 90 minutes. During this MedRAP orientation session, the PGY-1 residents are provided with important insight and tools for their first few weeks of residency.

The small group format facilitates communication among the new PGY-1 residents and allows them to ask questions they might be reluctant to bring up in the large group setting.

Organizational skills, in general, are the focus of the MedRAP program for the first two months because they are the most urgent skills to develop for effective navigation in the system. In these initial sessions, the PGY-1 residents are given some of the basic tools needed to help them function effectively, as quickly as possible, in residency.

Chapters 9 and 10 cover the details of the Orientation and Organizational Skills sessions.

MONTHS 3 – 6
Communication Skills Topics

Communication skills build residents' competencies in communicating with patients, patients' families, and the entire health care team. These sessions also assist in self-reflection about residents' own emotions and how they affect their interaction with others.

Chapters 11, 12, 13, and 14 cover the details of the Communication Skills sessions.

MONTHS 7 – 10
Quality Improvement / Management Skills

Months 7 through 10 focus on the QI component to improve management skills. Residents identify systemic errors in the different affiliated hospitals' work environments and use organizational techniques to come up with solutions, thus developing their management skills. The residents, along with the facilitator, prepare presentations that involve the entire health care team. This collaboration contributes to a more effective and efficient work environment, leading to positive organizational change.

Residents also evaluate their residency training program's strengths and weaknesses and meet with the program director in March to discuss suggested improvements.

Chapter 15 covers the details of the Quality Improvement and Management Skills sessions.

MONTHS 11 – 12
Leadership Skills Topics

Leadership skills are developed toward the end of the MedRAP program curriculum—which corresponds with the end of the academic year—because this is a point of transition for the PGY-1 residents. In preparation for their clinical team leadership responsibilities which commence in PGY-2, as well as the additional responsibilities that come with being second-year residents, the participants train for their leadership roles on both on an individual and organizational level.

Chapters 16 and 17 cover the details of the Leadership Skills sessions.

MONTH 12 OR 13
Annual Evaluation

In addition to the monthly evaluations conducted at every GL meeting, the facilitator conducts an annual needs assessment and analysis, distributing the MedRAP Residents' Annual Evaluation Questionnaire. The results help to formulate the subsequent year's session schedule, decide on the key topics to be covered, and incorporate new challenges the residents are likely to face. Since a significant part of the needs assessment is being conducted in the GLs' meeting, the facilitator can decide whether to conduct a separate evaluation session for PGY-1 residents in the beginning of June (month 13) or to distribute the evaluation forms at the end of the month 12 session. Chapter 18 covers the details of the Annual Evaluation and Planning session.

SESSION TOPICS	GOALS & OBJECTIVES	TOPICS
Orientation and Organizational Skills (Months 1 – 2)	• To help residents function more efficiently in the hospital work environment	• Orientation to internship year • Float call • Time management • Medical mistakes • Computer tips
Communication Skills (Months 3 – 6)	• To improve interaction with patients, their families, and health care professionals • To promote self-reflection processing skills that lead to more effective communication • To promote professionalism by developing sensitivity to cultural diversity and empathy	• Patient-physician interaction • Interaction with families • Breaking bad news • Communication with the health care team • Conflict resolution
Quality Improvement/ Management Skills (Months 7 – 10)	• To increase resident participation in health care quality improvement efforts • To assist in early identification of organizational problems • To develop problem solving methods utilized in industry • To improve collaboration with health care team • To contribute to future function of physicians	• Ongoing systematic collection of data • Organizational problem solving • Data analysis • Suggested solutions by residents • Presentation to management
Leadership Skills (Month 11-12)	• To prepare residents for future responsibilities as team leaders • To prepare residents for future leadership roles in the health care industry	• Strategies for senior residents • Leadership styles • Emotional intelligence (EQ) • Teaching tips • Effective evaluation
Ongoing and Annual Evaluation and Planning (Month 12 or 13)	• To conduct ongoing program evaluation in the monthly GLs meeting, ensuring PGY-1 needs are being met in sessions • To continue providing an effective response to residents' and management's needs	• Residents identify helpful components of the program, without worrying about communicating negative feedback to faculty who evaluate them

MEDRAP'S SESSIONS

MedRAP goes beyond the traditional support group model by merging it with a small group job training program, designed to formalize the informal training that occurs as the new residents interact with and learn from colleagues. The group format includes monthly meetings that aim to equip the new PGY-1 residents with tools to help them transition from medical school to residency. The meetings are led by a professional **facilitator** who is operationally independent from the residency program, and by senior resident **group leaders** (GLs) selected because of their perceived professionalism and ability to serve as effective role models. These GLs are identified as mentors by their peers, seniors, chiefs, and program management, and they also help tailor MedRAP materials for the monthly group sessions.

During these sessions, a mix of structured curriculum, interactive exercises, and group discussion is used to address each session's topic. The group members share experiences and self-reflect on issues related to the topic. GLs offer best practices, share experience-based tips, and review handouts prepared by the facilitator based on group members' feedback.

One of the MedRAP groups was comprised of Medicine Pediatric residents who were certified in both Internal Medicine and Pediatrics. They spent half of their time in the Internal Medicine department and half in the Pediatrics department. MedRAP developed a special curriculum for this group to consider the challenges they encountered in Internal Medicine and in Pediatrics departments. Their curriculum was tailored to address challenges they might encounter both with the adult population and with children and their families. They had special orientation sessions for their transition between the departments and a special quality control session designed especially for them. Their GLs were also Medicine Pediatric residents.

FACILITATOR ROLE

The MedRAP facilitator's role is to design and tailor the program to the evolving needs of the trainees, because conditions and needs change in both the residency program and the affiliated hospitals. The facilitator administers and facilitates the PGY-1 sessions with the help of the GLs.

Facilitator Roles:

- Conduct needs assessment
- Select and train GLs
- Collect feedback to identify session topics
- Design sessions
- Facilitate multiple PGY-1 groups based on departmental needs
- Collect ongoing feedback
- Provide individual assistance or referrals to residents experiencing problems
- Design and manage QI process for different affiliated hospitals
- Evaluate program effectiveness continuously
- Modify program based on feedback
- Communicate with management to address issues identified in ongoing feedback collection

Facilitating a MedRAP group of PGY-1 residents can be a challenging task. Residents come to the group meetings in one of the most difficult and busy years of their lives. In the PGY-1 year, they encounter many frustrations with the system, with managing their multiple clinical responsibilities, and with unmet expectations regarding their role as physicians.

Successful facilitators are:

- Of high intellectual caliber, with a graduate or post-graduate degree, able to earn the respect of participants
- Interested in organizational theory and techniques that foster constructive change
- Familiar with medical systems and medical terminology
- Highly empathetic
- Able to communicate in a diplomatic manner
- Skilled in conducting group work
- Operationally independent of the residency program

The fact that the facilitator is operationally independent from the residency program accelerates the PGY-1s' adaptation and professional development for several reasons:

- They are able to honestly share problems they experience with senior residents, faculty, or health care team members.
- The facilitator can address these problems with the chief residents or

program directors, leading to faster resolution and more effective functioning of the residents.

- Timely responses to reported issues contribute to a positive organizational culture.
- The safe environment also contributes to an accelerated learning curve because residents are able to share real concerns they have (for example, about making medical errors) and learn from their mistakes.
- Facilitators may be faculty members (see Mixed Faculty Model below) affiliated with the teaching institution but attending in other departments outside the residency program, thus retaining operational independence.
- If faculty members are utilized as group facilitators, they should sign a confidentiality agreement and serve as ombudsmen who would help ensure a safe environment and advocate for residents.

MIXED FACULTY MODEL CONSIDERATIONS

MedRAP achieves best results with facilitators who are independent of the residency program and well-versed in organizational, psychological, and medical terminology. The substantial return on investment justifies the allocation of resources. However, considering the economic constraints and limited resources faced by some medical institutions, the mixed faculty model is offered as an alternative. This model should be able to achieve most of the MedRAP goals if implemented as suggested. When considering facilitator candidates from a pool of the medical school faculty, it is important to ensure they can create and foster a safe environment for the group participants and serve as advocates for the residents. In order to achieve this operational independence, it is advisable to select faculty from other departments, such as Surgical faculty working with OBGYN residents or Internal Medicine faculty working with Pediatric residents. Mental health professionals with graduate or post-graduate degrees can work together with faculty in facilitating groups. The process for selecting faculty facilitators could be conducted by program directors, associate program directors, or the Graduate Medical Education committee within the institution.

The following criteria should be considered when selecting facilitators from a faculty pool:
- Interest in education of house staff
- Professionalism
- Team work capabilities
- Interest in constructive organizational change
- Competence
- Ability to empathize

- Ability to communicate constructively
- Skill in facilitating groups

The selection process would include:
- Identification of faculty members interested in trainee group facilitation
- Distribution of confidential questionnaires
- Selection of facilitators based on feedback

Incentives to faculty facilitators:
- Faculty facilitators could be relieved from their clinical responsibilities while facilitating groups and implementing the program, including conducting the needs analysis
- Facilitators could receive compensation and/or educational credit, contributing to opportunities for academic promotions

HIERARCHY OF CHOICES FOR FACILITATORS FOR OPTIMAL SAFE ENVIRONMENT

Facilitators could be completely independent of the institution, or operationally independent of the residency program but affiliated with the institution.

INDEPENDENT OF INSTITUTION
- Organizational psychologists
- Clinical psychologists
- Social workers
- MBAs with training in organizational behavior and management

MIXED FACULTY
- Medical school faculty from different departments who are operationally independent of the residency program, such as OBGYN faculty facilitating groups in the Internal Medicine Department

TWO FACILITATORS
- Groups can be led by 2 facilitators when utilizing the mixed faculty model
- For example, a faculty member who is operationally independent of the residency program could co-facilitate the groups with a mental health professional

OTHERS
- Mental health faculty in the institution
- Employee Assistance Program Counselors
- Human Service Counselors

GROUP LEADER ROLE

As mentioned before, MedRAP is designed to utilize senior residents as group leaders for the PGY-1 residents. Group leaders are carefully selected and trained to help lead the PGY-1 groups. This format has several advantages and benefits for the PGY-1 residents which include:

- Having an additional opportunity to further develop mentorship relationships
- Learning from the cumulative experiences of senior residents
- Sharing experiences and seeking personal advice from GLs in a confidential setting

Group Leader Role and Responsibilities:
- Monthly participation in GL session
- Help identify problems PGY-1s are likely to encounter
- Help tailor material to evolving PGY-1 needs
- Monthly participation in one assigned PGY-1 session
- Help lead PGY-1 session
- Provide individual assistance to PGY-1 if needed
- Help design and present QI presentation

Successful Group Leader Attributes:
- Effective ward team leader
- Professional in dealing with patients, colleagues, and health care team members
- Positive leadership skills
- Academically competent
- Motivated to help peers and subordinates
- Interested in bringing constructive change to the institution

Serving as a GL requires an investment of time and effort at a very busy time of the training. While GLs are generally self-motivated to help the PGY-1 residents, additional benefits and incentives, which can help them throughout their residency and beyond, include:

- Improvement of their leadership skills
- Learning techniques implemented in industry to improve organizational efficiency
- Participation in the QI presentations to residency program and affiliated hospitals' management, and being empowered to help bring constructive change

- An experience that can better prepare them for a chief resident role
- An opportunity to have their own peer support group in a confidential setting
- Serving in a leadership role that can be reflected in their recommendation letters and resumes and considered when they apply for chief resident roles, fellowships, and new jobs

MEDRAP'S SESSIONS STRUCTURE

Each month, facilitators run a **GL Session**, followed by the **PGY-1 Sessions**.

Group Leader Sessions

During GL Sessions, the content of the upcoming PGY-1 Session is discussed and determined, as well as concerns and challenges specific to the GL group. Facilitators lead discussions on the session topic, materials, and suggested improvements to existing handouts/activities/case studies. The GLs help identify the challenges the PGY-1 residents are likely to encounter relating to the specific session topic. They also self-reflect on their own experiences and brainstorm about best practices to handle the particular challenges.

GLs also provide feedback about their monthly experiences, which are different from the PGY-1 experiences. There are two reasons it's important for GLs to discuss their own experiences outside of PGY-1 sessions. First, separate GL sessions ensure that the PGY-1 sessions focus solely on PGY-1 issues. Secondly, separate sessions help identify problems and potential solutions specific to senior resident issues. Enabling senior residents to discuss their own challenges among their peers in a supportive community positively impacts their ability to function as effective GLs.

Objectives:
- To identify evolving needs of PGY-1 residents
- To identify typical challenges PGY-1s are likely to experience relating to the specific issues/topics
- To identify best practices and strategies relevant to each issue/topic
- To tailor the existing session materials for the residents' ongoing needs
- To address GLs' needs in a separate environment

GL Session Agenda:

Feedback	Confidential feedback is collected about GLs' experiences in their hospital rotations, which is often different from PGY-1 experiences. The issues they encounter are also addressed in the monthly meetings with residency program management. Feedback is reported anonymously to encourage honest disclosure without fear of repercussions.
Self-Reflection	GLs are given self-reflection exercises and questionnaires related to the topic of discussion to help analyze and break down components of problems they experience. GLs help identify typical challenges that PGY-1 residents are likely to encounter. This reflection is conducted through both written and oral feedback.
Review of Materials	Existing materials are analyzed and updated, including activities, tips, and best practices. Do these materials address the most important and challenging situations residents are likely to encounter?
Addition of Materials	GLs may have discovered tools as part of their informal training, practices that assisted them in their transition, or lessons that contributed to their professional development as residents. GLs assist facilitators in adding these tools to the curriculum.
Individual Assistance	Individual assistance is available to senior residents who experience personal or professional difficulties or want to discuss peers or colleagues they are concerned about (discussed in Chapter 7).

PGY-1 Sessions

The MedRAP PGY-1 sessions implement the curriculum that was updated and developed in the GL session. A small group format achieves multiple goals simultaneously, including creating a supportive environment and community, enhancing self-awareness, creating meaning and purpose at work, developing cognitive behavioral techniques to reframe negative experiences, and developing skills to facilitate effective transitions. These skills, environmental attributes, and activities have been reported to increase resilience, reduce burnout, and improve well-being in physicians.[1]

During the PGY-1 Sessions, challenges specific to residents are addressed through various strategies, such as self-reflection, activities, and discussion.

Objectives:

- To facilitate and accelerate transition from medical school to residency
- To develop organizational skills
- To develop interpersonal and communication skills
- To promote professionalism among residents
- To prepare residents for their future responsibilities as team leaders and other leadership roles in the health care industry
- To help residents identify their own leadership style
- To help the house staff develop problem-solving skills
- To assist them in early identification of organizational problems

PGY-1 Session Agenda:

Introduction	Introduction of topic and session objectives by facilitator
Feedback	Feedback collection on monthly rotation experiences and sharing of experiences with peers and senior residents; feedback from peers and GLs on best practices to handle challenging situations
Self-Reflection	Self-reflection activities related to topic of discussion (i.e. in organizational sessions, medical mistakes that PGY-1s commonly make; in communication sessions, challenging interactions with patients that elicit negative reactions)
Topic Experiential Exercises	Exercises to facilitate experiential learning related to session topic (i.e. case studies) • Discussion of cases and strategies to handle them with PGY-1 residents • GL input and additional suggested strategies
GL Input and Discussion	Discussion of handouts and general best practices suggested by the GLs and strategies prepared by the facilitators related to session topic
Conclusion	Summary of session goals and lessons learned
Individual Assistance	Individual assistance to residents experiencing personal or professional adjustment issues (conducted after the formal conclusion of the session)

MEDRAP'S ONGOING FEEDBACK MECHANISMS

MedRAP is a "living" program. Because of the constant feedback mechanisms inherent in the GL sessions, the PGY-1 sessions, and the end-of-year annual evaluation and planning sessions, the program constantly adjusts to residents' needs, as well as to changes in the training and work environment.

GROUP LEADER SESSION

Needs assessment with GLs

Describe typical
difficult situations

Identify the most
challenging problems

Identify best strategies

**FACILITATOR
MATERIAL PREPARATION**

Modify material
based on GL input

PGY-1 SESSIONS

Topic presented

Group discussion and exercises

Case Simulation,
Best Practices handouts

**FEEDBACK
FROM PARTICIPANTS**

Were the problems you
encountered addressed
by the session?

What can be done to improve?

Responses used to modify
material for following year

MEDRAP SESSION DESIGN PROCESS CREATES AN EVOLVING PROGRAM TO ADDRESS REAL VERSUS ASSUMED NEEDS

CHAPTER 5:

IMPLEMENTATION ROAD MAP

Before launching the MedRAP program, several pre-implementation steps are suggested to maximize the program's effectiveness. This chapter reviews each pre-implementation step in detail.

PRE-IMPLEMENTATION STEPS

3 MONTHS PRIOR TO INITIAL IMPLEMENTATION:
Conduct a Needs Analysis

1 MONTH PRIOR TO IMPLEMENTATION:
Select Group Leaders

1 MONTH PRIOR TO IMPLEMENTATION:
Create PGY-1 Groups

3 WEEKS PRIOR TO IMPLEMENTATION:
Conduct Group Leader Training

3 WEEKS PRIOR TO IMPLEMENTATION:
Tailor Program to Meet Real vs. Assumed Needs

CONDUCT A NEEDS ANALYSIS
3 months prior to initial implementation*

*Prior to each monthly topic session in subsequent years

Before designing any organizational intervention to deal with stress management, burnout reduction, or employee well-being improvement, and prior to prescribing any form of training, it is important to conduct a thorough needs assessment and organizational analysis to ensure the training program is addressing the stressors present in the target environment.

Although a set of stressors, such as the ones itemized in Chapter 3, may be common to residency, specific organizational stressors can vary by institution. Even within the same organization, stressors can differ from department to department, and the needs of employees in the same organization could change. Employees working in organizations are exposed to a wide range of challenges and situations that are potential stressors.

> Needs analysis is a useful technique that helps to identify the specific problems present in an organization. The needs analysis systematically breaks down problems and their individual components before drawing any conclusions. Using such an approach increases the likelihood of developing programs structured to deal with real, rather than assumed, needs.[1]

CONDUCTING AN EFFECTIVE NEEDS ASSESSMENT

In order to conduct an effective needs assessment in any organization, both work-related factors and individual-related factors should be identified.

Work-related stressors are divided into ***organizational stressors*** and ***individual stressors***. Both have long been recognized as being expensive because they take a toll both on the employee and on corporate health. Dysfunctional stress in organizations is associated with turnover, absenteeism, industrial accidents, and decline in the quantity and quality of production. Organizations, like individuals, can have distinct personalities. The personality of an organization is often shaped by its top executives and leadership and can often be a learned behavior among new employees.[2,3]

Organizational stressors include:

- An autocratic management team – This can create a culture of fear and cause other organizational stressors such as intra- and intergroup conflict.
- Poor relationships within and between groups in the organization – These may result in low levels of trust, lack of cohesion or sense of support, and lack of interest in identifying and dealing with problems.
- Inadequate employee participation – This limits the extent to which a

person's knowledge, opinions, and ideas are included in the decision-making process. Organizations that do not allow or encourage participation can be a source of frustration for those who value it.

> A stressor is a demand made by the internal or external environment that upsets a person's balance and for which restoration is needed.

- Lack of performance feedback – Employees want to know how they are doing and how their superiors view their work. Lacking constructive performance evaluation feedback or receiving it in a highly critical manner can create stress in the employee. In order to minimize stress, performance feedback should be an open, two-way communication system.

Individual stressors include:

- Role conflict – How an individual behaves in any given situation depends in large part on the demands and expectations he places on himself versus those placed on him by others. Role conflict arises when one set of these demands and expectations makes it difficult to comply with another.
- Role ambiguity – This results from a lack of clarity about the job objectives and the job responsibilities. Chronic ambiguity can elicit a stress response that can be negative and maladaptive in nature and poses a threat to the employees' adaptation.
- Work overload – Quantitative work overload occurs when a worker has too many things to do and not enough time to do them. Qualitative overload occurs when the worker feels he does not have the ability to do his job or cannot perform his job at the expected level, no matter how much time he might have to complete it. If this feeling is chronic, it may affect the quality of decision-making and inter-personal relationships, leading to costly and dangerous mistakes.

In order to conduct an effective organizational assessment, two forms of needs analysis—that coincide with the two types of stressors—are essential:

Organizational Analysis

The organizational analysis should determine what is causing or contributing to difficulties and areas that employees are reporting to be a problem. Both employee and management input are needed for an informative and accurate organizational needs analysis. It is important that top management be supportive of the training and be aware of what objectives the training program is attempting to achieve. The following questions should be addressed:

- What are the main producers of stress in the organization?
- Do they detract from the attainment of organizational goals?
- Is it possible to alleviate them through a training program?
- How can its effectiveness be evaluated?
- What are the specific goals of the training program?

Individual Analysis

An individual analysis should provide specific clues about the difficulties individual employees are experiencing. Deficiencies can be due to lack of knowledge or skills, a poor attitude, or unmanaged stress on or off the job. An individual analysis should be combined with the organizational analysis data. Each analysis provides different sets of data. The organizational stress-induced problems can impact individuals in different ways. Both can be addressed in a well-designed stress management training program. When deficiencies or problems are identified, the cause or reason should be uncovered. The following questions should be addressed:

- What are the prevalent difficulties individual residents are experiencing?
- Will the individual benefit from some form of training in order to best perform in the organization?
- What knowledge will be useful for the transition?
- What skills can be developed to assist in areas of struggle?

PROGRAM SESSION DESIGN

The overall MedRAP program structure addresses the stressors identified in the initial needs analysis. Several parts of the MedRAP structure help address both organizational and individual stressors. Some parts constitute the overarching themes of the program and make up the backbone of the MedRAP system; these include creating a safe environment to collect anonymous feedback and to self-reflect, and empowering residents to participate in improving their training and work environment. Other parts, such as the topics for individual sessions, can be modified according to a hospital's individual needs assessment.

INITIAL NEEDS ANALYSIS AT THE DEPARTMENT OF INTERNAL MEDICINE AT BCM

The initial needs analysis for the MedRAP program was a two-phase process that included an organizational analysis and an individual analysis. They both formed the basis for the program design. Please note that, although a needs analysis was conducted every year to update the session topics, strategies to deal with challenges, and materials, the thorough analysis as described below was only conducted during the first year.

At BCM, this initial needs analysis uncovered the stressors as discussed in Chapter 3, upon which the BCM MedRAP program was based. Any medical institution can implement a similar needs analysis to identify their own unique stressors.

PHASE I: IDENTIFYING PROBLEMS

- Organizational analysis included:
  - ◉ Meetings with small groups of residents, chief residents, and faculty to identify general causes of difficulties during first year of residency
  - ◉ Based on feedback, development of questionnaires to administer to larger groups to validate information
  - ◉ Administration of questionnaires to large groups of residents to identify common issues
- Individual analysis included:
  - ◉ Individual interviews to identify individual residents' needs and recognize common themes
  - ◉ Exercise to identify individual stressors (For example, a short film, presenting 30 different stressful situations that PGY-1 residents may encounter, was viewed during the BCM needs analysis, and the residents then identified the ones that were relevant to them.)[4]
  - ◉ Identification of common themes in the individual stressors reported

PHASE II: IDENTIFYING WAYS TO ADDRESS THE PROBLEMS

- Small groups of three or four senior residents offered their perception of the most effective ways to address the difficulties identified in the first stage. (Organizational analysis)
- Based on their cumulative experiences, they identified those personal attributes and skills that would have helped them most throughout their first year of residency. (Individual analysis)
- Residents revealed their preferred remedy modes, which included problem-solving approaches, case studies, and group discussions, rather than role-playing and various relaxation techniques.

Figure I: The MedRAP Needs Analysis Design Process

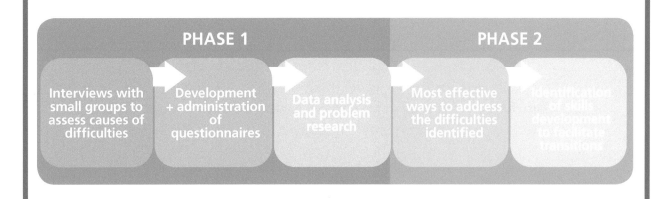

SELECT GROUP LEADERS
1 month prior to implementation

In order to create more opportunities for mentorship, facilitate the transfer of collective wisdom, and formalize informal training, senior residents were selected as Group Leaders (GLs) through a specially designed process, considering input from:

- PGY-1 residents
- Senior residents
- Chief residents
- Program director

Selection criteria included:

- Leadership skills
- Perceived professionalism
- Efficiency as a PGY-1 or PGY-2 resident
- Academic performance
- Performance in teams (i.e. willingness to help peers)

Three senior residents were assigned as GLs to each PGY-1 group: two second-year senior residents and one third-year. The rationale was that the second-year GLs were closer to the internship year and thus more familiar with problems and strategies specific to this year. The hospital system, the training experience, and expectations continuously change. The second-year GLs equipped the PGY-1s with tips and tools to help them function more effectively. The third-year resident would add a broader perspective about the residency experience and planning for the future. Also, as the Department of Medicine residency program at BCM was structured, the second-year residents served as ward team leaders on only one of the affiliated hospital's systems and were more familiar with the work environment there, while the third-year residents served as ward team leaders in the other affiliated hospital and were more familiar with its system.

Part of the GL selection process included demographic considerations that reflected the diversity of the PGY-1 groups. Factoring in demographic considerations contributed to the function of the group. Some of the PGY-1s seemed to identify better with role models from similar backgrounds/cultures. It also assisted the PGY-1s' professional development, as they were exposed to different cultures and had an opportunity to learn about them from their different mentors.

CREATE PGY-1 GROUPS
1 month prior to implementation

MedRAP factored in demographic considerations when creating the PGY-1 groups, reflecting the diversity of the PGY-1 class. This heterogeneous grouping helped facilitate understanding and sensitivity to each other, leading to a more supportive training environment. It also allowed the PGY-1 residents to learn from each other about cultural differences and considerations when taking care of patients. Every group included several BCM graduates, enabling PGY-1 residents from other parts of the country, as well as International Medical Graduates (IMGs), to learn about the BCM system from them. Doing so also helped to better integrate residents from other places into the residency program, creating a more cohesive group. The facilitator carefully designed the PGY-1 sessions by factoring in GL feedback to maximize effectiveness.

New PGY-1 residents came to the MedRAP sessions with a variety of individual differences. The overall MedRAP program structure addresses the stressors identified in the initial needs analysis. It is important to create a positive and supportive environment to improve relationships in the group and residency. To foster such relationships among the PGY-1 groups, the following guidelines were established:

- In this training program, professionalism is defined not only by how they treat their patients, but also by how they treat each other.
- The meetings are completely confidential due to the fact that the facilitator operates independently of the residency program.
- Should participants experience a problem requiring external intervention from program management, their consent will be obtained prior to any sharing of information.
- The facilitator and group leaders are always available to assist, including outside of the group setting.
- PGY-1 residents come to the group from different parts of the country, different cultures, and with different needs.
    - At times, you may feel that a segment of the program is not answering your particular needs. Remember that someone else's needs are currently being met, even if yours are not.

GROUP STRUCTURE

- Balanced mix of male and female PGY-1 residents
- Several graduates from the medical school affiliated with the residency program
- Graduates from other medical schools in the country
- International medical graduates

⊙   There might be other times when your needs will be addressed, rather than someone else's.

⊙   We are here to help each other; the objective is that, while participants enter the group as individuals, they will support each other and leave the session as a cohesive group.

CONDUCT GROUP LEADER TRAINING
3 weeks prior to implementation

The first GL session was dedicated to training the senior residents and providing tools to optimize their leadership in MedRAP groups. The session highlighted the differences between being a group participant and group leader. They reflected back to their own GLs and identified reasons they found them to be helpful and why. Then they identified their potential strengths and weaknesses as GLs. The residents then received a few additional tips to help them lead, some of which included:

- **Foster a professional environment where:**
  - ⊙   Everyone is treated with respect even during a disagreement;
  - ⊙   It is safe for differences to be expressed;
  - ⊙   Differences and difficulties are dealt with in a constructive manner.
- **Listen carefully:** Focus on listening rather than being concerned about what to say next. Participants' ideas and thoughts are the best source of follow-up questions and comments. Listening intently also sends a message that participants' thoughts are valuable.
- **Get everyone to contribute:** Make it a point to address questions to those who speak rarely or not at all. Do not let a few articulate members dominate the discussion.
- **Ask follow-up questions:** Many times, participants do not say exactly what they mean or offer what appear to be superficial comments. Ask one or more follow-up questions to help participants articulate their ideas more clearly. Follow-up questions are also your "contact" with your group. Your questions keep participants attentive and help them focus on the central problem.
- **Be a role model:** The goal of these training sessions is to create a professional environment where everyone participates and shares experiences in a nonjudgmental and respectful manner, even when there is disagreement. It is the GL's responsibility to:
  - ⊙   Foster an atmosphere in the groups that will be carried out to the wards;

⊙ Model behavior in the groups that you would want to see replicated outside the group;

⊙ Listen nonjudgmentally and use what you hear in a constructive manner.

TAILOR PROGRAM TO MEET REAL VS. ASSUMED NEEDS
3 weeks prior to implementation

Annually, GLs review with the facilitator the previous year's session topics, goals, and materials in the first group leaders' meeting, analyzing which session topics are still relevant and applicable to the needs of future incoming PGY-1 residents. Program management's recommendations are also considered. New materials are also developed prior to every topic session to make sure the information is current.

It is important to note that MedRAP's curriculum is continuously tailored to meet the emerging needs of both residents and management. Continuous needs assessment is a key component of the program. Although the initial material for the program can be based on a one-time analysis, it is only through ongoing needs analysis and participants' feedback collection that the program can continuously meet residents' and management's needs.

Due to its commitment to ongoing needs assessment, MedRAP constantly evolves. Because of this, it remains a consistently useful program for professional development and an effective mechanism to bring constructive organizational change. The program continually offers revised materials and added (or dropped) sessions as the residency program and the hospital work environment changes. The continuous adaptation to the training and work environment, tailoring it to residents' real rather than assumed needs, is instrumental to any training program's longevity and success.

MedRAP is most effective and impactful when implemented as designed, utilizing a small group format led by facilitators and senior resident group leaders who are selected for their professionalism and teamwork capabilities.

In situations where this program structure cannot be fully applied, individual residents can still benefit from the provided strategies, tips, and tools to help prepare them to meet the challenges they are likely to encounter.

SECTION 3

STRUCTURAL COMPONENTS

Along with session-specific activities, every MedRAP session includes three core components that are fundamental to the program's structure:

- Collection of anonymous feedback
- Time for individual assistance
- Mechanisms to facilitate organizational professionalism

Collectively, these components contribute to overall program effectiveness by fostering a safe environment, which leads to a constructive and positive organizational culture. The next three chapters describe these components and provide guidelines on how to implement and incorporate them in the sessions.

CHAPTER 6:
COLLECTING CONFIDENTIAL FEEDBACK

The American Medical Association (AMA) emphasizes the importance of collecting ongoing feedback in its Practice Transformation series: *Burnout. 2015.*[1] To facilitate open communication associated with burnout reduction, the AMA suggests providing a mechanism for health care providers to give ongoing feedback, improve communication, and facilitate flow of information upwards to the top levels of management. They also feel it is possible to accelerate learning while sharing and communicating experiences and problems to management, leading to better collaboration with leadership on an ongoing basis. Some methods can include:

- Setting aside dedicated time to share concerns
- Holding office hours with leaders to allow feedback
- Putting out a comment box for anonymous feedback
- Sharing challenging patient case studies

Communication is essential to the success of effective organizations, and it is recommended that any effective organization should facilitate communication in four distinct directions: downward, upward, horizontally, and diagonally.[2]

Downward communication: flows from individuals in higher levels of the organization's hierarchy to those in lower levels.

Upward communication: flows from the individual at lower levels of the organizational structure to those at higher levels.

Horizontal communication: flows across functions in the organization (i.e., between different departments or different units of the organization).

Diagonal communication: cuts across functions and levels in the organization; important in situations where members cannot communicate effectively through traditional channels and bypassing it would be most efficient in terms of time and effort in the organization.

Feedback is defined as the act of providing knowledge of the results of behavior or performance to the individual. In the health care industry, specifically, feedback is described as, "Any summary of clinical performance of health care over a specified period of time, given in a written, electronic or verbal format." In addition, feedback is, "An informed, non-evaluative, objective appraisal of performance intended to improve clinical skills." Feedback should incorporate some action to close the identified gap and promote improvement. From an organizational standpoint, consistent feedback over time can be an important mechanism for organizational learning, resulting in both "Incremental and large-scale modification to care systems and processes."[3]

Effective communication and collaboration in health care is achieved when health care professionals work together cooperatively, sharing responsibilities in order to make decisions to formulate and carry out plans for patient care.[4] Collaboration among the health care team increases their awareness of each other's specific knowledge, roles, and abilities, leading to improved decision-making.[4]

Components of Facilitating Successful Communication:

- Safe and non-punitive environment
- Respectful, constructive atmosphere
- Specific roles and tasks for all team members
- Acknowledgment and processing of conflict
- Clear and known channels to handle the feedback
- Regular and routine communication and information sharing
- Mechanism to evaluate outcomes and adjust accordingly

An effective communication system improves information flow, leading to more effective and safe interventions. It also contributes to improved employee morale, better quality of care, patient and family satisfaction, and shorter hospital stays.[4]

Health professionals tend to work independently and autonomously, even though they work as part of a team. Communication and collaboration barriers that exist between clinical staff can impact efforts to improve health care safety and quality. Barriers to effective communication among health care professionals include organizational, psychological, and educational factors and have some common themes.[5,6]

Common Barriers to Health Care Professionals' Communication and Collaboration:

- Personality differences and individualism
- Differences in culture and ethnicity
- Generational differences
- Differences in schedules and professional routines
- Differences in requirements, regulations, and norms of professional education
- Differences in accountability, payment, and rewards
- Concerns regarding clinical responsibility
- Personal values and expectations
- Hierarchy
- Complexity of care
- Emphasis on rapid decision making

Relationships among health care professionals providing patient care can have a powerful influence on how and if important information is communicated. Poor health care team communication can delay patient care. Research suggests that clinicians need standardized communication tools because of the intrinsic limitations of human performance and the complexity of patient care.[5] An optimal hospital organizational environment encourages individuals to speak openly and express concerns.[7]

Creating opportunities for different groups to meet and share experiences is a highly effective strategy for enhancing collaboration and communication. Group meetings encourage open dialogue and frequently provide an upfront solution that reduces the likelihood of systemic errors. Besides maintaining confidentiality and reducing risks of retaliation, one of the most crucial aspects of the feedback collection is to give assurance that identified complaints and problems will be addressed, and appropriate actions will be taken. Responses should be timely, consistent, and provide necessary feedback and follow-up.

Effective medical practice must also focus on increasing opportunities for communication and collaboration, thereby accelerating early identification and solution of organizational problems. In order to enhance clinical outcomes, it is important for health care organizations to offer programs to help foster honest and constructive communication across the organization.

Ongoing clinical feedback is an important component of the development and education of medical trainees, contributing to their competence and confidence.[3] Feedback collection should be conducted regularly, and participation of all trainees is encouraged as an integral, ongoing and consistent aspect of a physician's education and training. Young physicians can use feedback opportunities to reflect on their experiences, enhance personal development, and improve patient care.

BENEFITS OF COLLECTING ACCURATE FEEDBACK

One of the first things identified in the MedRAP BCM needs assessment was that the residents felt there was no place they could provide honest feedback because of their concerns about future implications and retribution. A large discrepancy emerged between the information reported during formal evaluation departmental meetings, versus the information communicated to the independent facilitator. Substantial important information, related to both resident training experiences and patient care, was not being conveyed to residency program management. The residents were worried about reporting problems they experienced with different members of the health care team, such as their senior residents, faculty, and nursing staff on the wards. They felt it could impact their monthly evaluations, call schedule, or assistance from the nursing staff, which is imperative to junior doctors. Even if they made a complaint through the appropriate channel and communicated concerns, they worried about repercussions. Clearly, an effective mechanism to collect the feedback in a safe environment would have the following specific benefits:

- It would assist with the early identification and solution of problems that PGY-1 residents experienced on the ward through:
  - Sharing challenges with peers, mentors and facilitator, and brainstorming on best strategies and practices that would prepare them to handle the challenge, hopefully, ahead of time
  - Receiving individual assistance from group leaders or facilitator related to personal difficulties
  - Having the independent facilitator maintain confidentiality while communicating the problem to chief residents and program director in an attempt to find solutions
- It would help create a positive, non-judgmental, and safe environment associated with improved well-being and morale, and reduced levels of burnout.
- It would accelerate flow of information to management regarding:
  - Systemic issues in the hospital work environment and general efficiency
  - Function of different health care team members
  - General morale issues
- It would help identify individual difficulties early--both educational and personal--allowing for subsequent follow-up.

- It would empower the PGY-1 residents, allowing them to be part of the identification and resolution of issues related to their training or work environment, giving them a valuable opportunity to impact the system.
- It would facilitate learning from each other and set realistic expectations for future rotations. The PGY-1 residents would have an opportunity to ask questions about rotations, and what aspects require the greatest attention (i.e., hierarchy, communication preferences of the attending physician, special tips particular to the service that can help accelerate patient care). PGY-1 residents would learn specific tips and would be provided with tools to be efficient on the future rotation. These discussions would also rely on the seniors' "institutional memory" and accelerate the learning curve for the PGY-1 residents, thus facilitating the transfer of specific collective wisdom and formalizing useful informal training.
- It would lead to early identification of problems and solutions related to patient care, positively impacting patients' satisfaction.

MEDRAP'S APPROACH TO COLLECTING FEEDBACK

MedRAP's Safe Environment Factor (SEF) is described as the condition created when residents feel free to express concerns, vulnerabilities, and any negative feelings, and to share medical mistakes in an environment that does not impact their standing in the residency program. The learning curve is accelerated as a result of maintaining the SEF, so that residents are able to openly share concerns with others who have had similar experiences.

One of the ways MedRAP shows residents they are in a safe environment is by collecting repercussion-free feedback. MedRAP facilitators collect feedback at three specific points in the program:

1. **Initial needs assessment** identifies problems in the upward and horizontal communication channels. The needs assessment is covered in detail in Chapter 5.

2. **Session feedback** addresses upward communication challenges. This feedback is collected at the beginning of each session. Residents report educational and organizational problems experienced in their rotations. The safe environment contributes to more honest and open feedback. The facilitator, maintaining resident anonymity, communicates the feedback to the program director and chief residents. This accelerates the flow of information and is instrumental in the early identification and solution of problems. This ongoing feedback collection can transmit information more rapidly than the formal system. The group participants also offer solutions to problems identified, which is empowering and keeps the

constructive orientation of the session. Successful organizations involve staff in finding solutions.[8]

3. **Annual quality improvement (QI)** addresses horizontal communication challenges. Questionnaires are developed to identify strengths and weaknesses within the hospital environments and the residency program. The data regarding each training hospital's work environment is analyzed to highlight the most important issues affecting patient care. Residents then develop realistic solutions to propose to the health care team. Group leaders are trained to present these solutions in a systematic and constructive way. The data regarding residency training is gathered and analyzed in the same manner and presented at a special annual meeting with the program director. The discussions and open exchange of ideas that follow all QI presentations lead to improvements in the training and hospital environments (discussed in Chapter 15).

TIPS FOR COLLECTING ONGOING FEEDBACK

- Group leaders provide feedback in a separate session to utilize time efficiently and to maintain perception of GLs as constructive.
- Dedicate about 15- 20 minutes to feedback collection.
- If an individual resident is upset, seems like he is struggling, or is taking too long, ask him to stay to discuss the issue after the session.
- Assign one GL to record issues reported. It is important that the facilitator maintain eye contact and observe nonverbal communication with the resident and in the group.
- Having the GL report helps to improve understanding of the issue by the facilitator as well, so they can go over it after the session.
- Develop a form that can facilitate recording of feedback (i.e., problem, components, suggested solutions).
- It is helpful to bring the completed form to the other group sessions to identify if a problem is viewed as a trend or has to do with a personal difficulty.
- Try to end on a positive note even if the feedback is negative (i.e., *I realize there are many weaknesses to this rotation; are there any strengths? Things you learned?*).
- Try to identify solutions to a problem experienced; involve group and GLs in brainstorming. Having the group generate solutions is empowering.
- All of the groups' feedback, including the GLs' feedback, is summarized and presented in monthly meetings with the program director. Before the meeting, feedback is analyzed, prioritized, and consolidated to identify the most important issues, patterns, trends, and areas for improvements. Minor issues requiring immediate attention are presented to the chief residents.
- If anonymity is important to a PGY-1 resident, assess the problem's prevalence and present it later as a concern shared collectively by the group.
- Acute issues that involve suboptimal patient care or physician's function need to be addressed promptly (i.e., harassment, abuse, patient safety). Acute issues tend to be addressed more openly. In that case, resident's permission should be obtained. These are addressed immediately by approaching the program director as needed, rather than waiting for the monthly meeting.

CHAPTER 7:

INDIVIDUAL ASSISTANCE

Residency training is well known for producing physical and mental stress in medical residents. They can experience a wide variety of professional and personal difficulties. About 8-15% of residents are estimated to have serious problems, presenting a special challenge for residency programs. Approximately 20% of program directors report avoidance issues related to "problem residents", fearing legal retribution. Residents are often reluctant to communicate difficulties because of the implications for their future, such as licensure issues, competency and milestone evaluations, and applications for fellowships or future jobs.[1]

The American Board of Internal Medicine's (ABIM) definition of a problem resident is: "A trainee who demonstrates a significant enough problem that requires intervention by someone of authority, usually the program director or chief resident."[1] The ABIM relies on residency programs to evaluate residents' competence and readiness to be eligible for graduating from residency programs; thus, there are different ways training programs attempt to standardize resident evaluation. Following the identification of a problem resident, program directors often have to help facilitate the successful remedy of the problem. Only when the problem is resolved can they recommend the resident for promotion, graduation, and certification.

Common stressors during residency fall into three categories:

1. Situational stressors: inordinate hours; sleep deprivation; excessive work load; overbearing paper work; dealing with electronic medical records; high risk patients; and conditions for learning that are less than optimal.

2. Personal stressors: family (may be a source of support and/or of conflict and stress); debts and financial issues; limited free time to relax or

socialize; underlying psychosocial issues highlighted due to residency stress; and inadequate coping skills.

3. Professional stressors: responsibility for patient care; challenging interactions with superiors, peers, subordinates, or members of the health care team, such as nurses; supervision responsibilities; difficult interactions with patients and their families; and career planning.

All of these factors can impact a resident's performance, and each resident reacts differently depending on that individual's coping mechanism.

Residency programs employ significant resources in recruiting and evaluating applicants to their training programs. Most applicants will become successful residents who will graduate without interruption. But not all residents will thrive; some trainees will fall below minimal performance standards, and their behaviors will interfere with their adjustment and function. Residency programs often fail to predict which trainees will experience problems, in spite of careful selection processes.

Problem residents can significantly impact the entire residency program, especially in cases where they are unable to continue performing their clinical duties. Measures must be taken to protect patients' care, and these steps often impact resources of other residents and faculty. At times, disciplinary actions require legal consultation, and remediation plans can result in time spent by faculty in monitoring, counseling, and evaluating the problem resident. Problem residents can also impact morale in the residency training program. Identifying problem residents and predicting poor performance presents a great challenge for residency programs; therefore, it is very important to accurately identify and address problems in a timely manner, before situations escalate. Once identified, problems may be resolved rapidly, may require remediation and disciplinary actions, or can result in failure to successfully complete training. Regardless, it is important to establish mechanisms in the residency training program to manage the problem effectively and minimize negative consequences.

Because peers and colleagues spend the most time with each other, they are often in the best position to detect impairment. However, house staff do not always feel comfortable confronting their colleagues, and don't always know how to do it in a supportive way. They are often reluctant to notify the chief residents or program director because they worry about consequences to the resident. Settings such as support groups—where residents can reflect on self-awareness and self-care—can be beneficial for early detection and prevention of problems, if conducted in a safe environment. Underlying causes that may contribute to poor performance are:

- Difficulty coping with stress
- Behavioral issues related to professionalism
- Medical conditions, including psychiatric illness
- Substance abuse
- Cultural differences
- Cognitive issues such as inadequate knowledge base or learning disabilities

Depression and emotional impairment are quite common in residency.[1] About one third of residents are reported to suffer from depression or psychological distress during internship. Only a few depressed PGY-1 residents consult mental health professionals. Residents worry about the future implications of seeking help from a psychiatrist, even if their counseling sessions are free. Off-campus counseling can reassure the resident that confidentiality will be maintained.[1] As discussed before, physicians as a group experience higher rates of emotional exhaustion and depression, as well as alcoholism, drug abuse, troubled marriages, divorce, and suicide. In general, physicians are reluctant to seek help, either from each other--because of confidentiality issues or future implications--or from a Physicians Health Program (PHP), fearing the power of medical boards and their ability to impact physicians' future careers.[2]

Residency programs attempt to identify and assist problem residents through:

- Feedback and discussion of concerns
- Advisor/advisee system
- Support groups among residents
- Planned social events, retreats
- Changing the schedule of highly-stressed residents
- Promotion of self-awareness and self-care

The first year of residency is often the most stressful period in the medical profession.[3] A successful residents' professional development training program can reduce stress for residents as a group, facilitate an optimal environment for their professional growth and their long-term well-being, facilitate successful conflict resolution, and assure the protection and safety of patients.

THE PSYCHOLOGY OF INDIVIDUAL DIFFERENCES WHEN DEALING WITH PROFESSIONAL ADJUSTMENT ISSUES

When helping residents adjust to their working environment, it is important to remember that they differ in their ability to handle stressful situations. In helping individual residents with professional adjustment issues, the traits and characteristics that distinguish them from one another should be considered. While individual assistance should be tailored to the resident and the particular difficulties experienced, it is helpful to recognize common themes and difficulties. Much of what makes up a person's way of seeing and responding to the world is a result of environmental factors, such as prior experiences and previous learning. From the perspective of the organization, it's important to have an understanding of how these differences affect individuals in order to minimize dysfunctional stress.[4,5]

Individual differences affect:
- How they make decisions
- How they handle conflict
- How they respond to and attempt to cope with stress
- Whether or not a stressor will be perceived as stressful
- Various outcomes that result from individuals reacting to the same stressor

Outcomes can be:
- Physiological
- Psychological
- Behavioral

Differences between people that can affect these outcomes are in the area of:
- Perception of control
- Responsibility
- Social support

Example: The health and performance consequences that follow those stress outcomes are similarly affected by individual differences. One resident experiencing a great deal of stress may make numerous errors as a result of that stress, while another may not make any errors but will frequently be late or absent from their shift.

Some of the individual differences associated with environmentally-shaped attributes impacting stress can be categorized as cognitive/affective. These attributes are also thought of as aspects of personality. There are four important characteristics of this category:[4]

- **Tolerance for ambiguity** appears to be an important individual difference affecting the stress experience. PGY-1 residents work in different environments under the supervision of different team leaders. For example: some leaders create a more structured environment than others; thus, PGY-1s with a high need for structure (a low tolerance for ambiguity and especially role ambiguity) will function better in these environments because it lessens the likelihood that it will be seen as threatening, and it will increase their capability to deal effectively with stress. On the other hand, PGY-1s with a high tolerance for ambiguity may find that a highly structured environment increases stress. Such a PGY-1 would welcome the stimulation and challenge associated with a situation of uncertainty.

- **Locus of control** refers to beliefs individuals have as to where control over their lives resides. They are either internals, who believe they are in control of the events that shape their lives, or externals, who feel that control is external to them. Typically, internals are less likely to be stressed because they believe that they can control what happens to them, while externals can often feel helpless and stressed. At times, however, internals may experience stress when they are unable to control a situation, while externals will feel especially stressed when they are put in a situation in which they do have the capability to exercise some control over events.

- **Self-esteem** and the relationship with stress is a significant one. People with high levels of self-esteem are confident in their abilities and generally feel good about themselves. They are less likely to feel threatened, but when they do, they are more likely to deal with the threat quickly, effectively, and with minimal dysfunctional outcomes and consequences. Self-esteem also plays a part in the perception of stressors. PGY-1s with low self-esteem are more likely to experience qualitative and quantitative overload.

- **Hardiness** is a "positive" individual difference that reduces the likelihood of stress and minimizes the incidence and severity of dysfunctional outcomes and consequences. It determines who stays healthy under stress, as opposed to who gets sick from stress. Three things that are important when dealing effectively with stress are:

  - A sense of commitment to various aspects of one's life; a sense of purpose and active involvement in life

  - The belief that one is in control of his life; the ability to respond to and transform potentially negative situations

  - Actively seeking out novelty and challenge, as opposed to familiarity and security

In summary, it is not stressors that produce stress; it is the significance, meaning, and interpretation that individuals assign to stressors. That interpretation is determined by individual differences. What is important is how these differences moderate stress, knowledge of individuals with respect to these differences, and action based on this knowledge. It is important to address these individual differences while helping residents adjust to their work environment.[6]

MEDRAP'S APPROACH TO PROVIDING INDIVIDUAL ASSISTANCE

The MedRAP program incorporates individual assistance into its format with the goal of facilitating early detection and prevention of problems. During the first session, PGY-1 residents are told that time will be allocated at the end of every session for individual assistance. They are assured of confidentiality by the fact that the facilitator is a professional who is operationally independent of the residency program.

The senior residents are trained to: (1) Identify PGY-1 residents or students experiencing problems; (2) Approach them in a confidential manner; (3) Help them identify the underlying issues; and (4) Identify possible solutions and help them cope. The PGY-1 residents are provided with this same training at the end of their internship year (see Chapters 16 and 17). They are also asked to be alert to their peers and subordinates, and to notify the facilitator if they think a colleague is experiencing difficulties and needs help.

The facilitator initiates meetings in the following situations:

- A resident is observed, during the meeting, to be experiencing difficulties.
- A senior resident group leader alerts the facilitator to difficulties individuals are experiencing.
- A peer resident alerts the facilitator to difficulties individuals are experiencing.
- The program director or chiefs are concerned about the function of a resident.
- The resident evaluation committee requests the facilitator to meet with a particular resident.
- Residents do not show up to the majority of meetings.

Personal problems experienced by residents could be due to:

- Professional adjustment issues (i.e., inefficiency, poor communication with health care team, trouble dealing with authority figures)
- Personal difficulties or problems (i.e., dealing with relationships outside the residency program, depressive tendencies, substance abuse)

Depending on the scope and severity of a resident's problem, assistance could be limited to one post-session meeting, or encompass several meetings in the facilitator's office to provide strategic planning to effectively deal with the difficulties.

Strategies for professional adjustment issues:

- Meeting/s with facilitator utilizing problem-solving, cognitive, communication, and conflict resolution techniques
- Facilitating confidential individual mentorship instruction (time management, efficiency) with one of the GLs
- The facilitator addressing more urgent issues confidentially with chiefs or program director
- The facilitator identifying more serious underlying issues and referring the resident for more assistance, either within or outside the institution

Strategies for personal difficulties:

- Identifying the cause of the problem
- Addressing mild, less serious issues with the resident in one or several meetings
- Referring residents to the house staff psychiatrist service for more acute serious issues (the residents at BCM had 10 free sessions); establishing a personal relationship between the facilitator and the house staff psychiatrist can ensure prompt access if needed
- Providing a list of available mental health clinicians to residents resistant to receiving help within the institution, due to confidentiality issues

The list was compiled with the help of one of the psychiatric department faculty. Consistent follow-up ensured the resident was actually getting help, and the mental health clinicians communicated, when needed, with the facilitator.

CHAPTER 8:

PERSONAL AND ORGANIZATIONAL PROFESSIONALISM

The professionalism of physicians has been widely discussed and defined, and its decline has been described as a public health issue.[1-3] However, the professionalism of health care organizations has only recently been systematically described in greater detail.[4]

IMPACT OF ORGANIZATIONAL PROFESSIONALISM ON PHYSICIANS' PERSONAL PROFESSIONALISM

Creating an environment of both personal and organizational professionalism is challenging, but just as personal well-being creates resiliency, health care organizations can establish mechanisms that buffer internal and external stressors. Establishing preventative measures can contribute to a positive organizational culture, thereby contributing to overall organizational professionalism.[5-7]

Significant resources have been directed towards the reduction of preventable diagnostic patient injuries. However, recent research suggests that these are more likely to occur in an environment where acceptable behaviors are not clearly enforced, and organizational professionalism is not embraced. An unprofessional organizational culture can contribute to suboptimal patient care.[4,6,8]

Leadership is critically important to establishing an atmosphere of professionalism in health care organizations. The leaders of the organization should be committed to establishing and maintaining a framework for direct communication, which promotes collaboration among the staff and the health care team, and contributes to correcting systemic problems and improving patient care. Positive interpersonal relationships should be cultivated through direct communication with the staff, solicitation of feedback, transparency about organizational goals, issues and initiatives, and support of organizational values.[9]

Additionally, organizational leaders can foster personal professionalism by maintaining a culture of safety, trust, and quality throughout the hospital. They must create environments in which physicians and other health care professionals are able to express their capacity for high-quality, compassionate care, while discouraging behaviors which negatively affect coworker communication,

PERSONAL PROFESSIONALISM VS. ORGANIZATIONAL PROFESSIONALISM

Personal Professionalism: ACGME defines physician professionalism as commitment to high standards of professional conduct, demonstrating altruism, compassion, honesty and integrity; adherence to principles of ethics and confidentiality; and consideration of religious, ethnic, gender, educational and other differences in interacting with patients and other members of the health care team.

Organizational Professionalism: Professional health care organizations are described as organizations whose culture upholds ethical values similar to those expected from individual physicians, such as beneficence, dignity, justice, honesty, and self-discipline. The organization has both formal and informal policies that support these values and create a positive organizational culture. Such an environment facilitates optimal professional development of individual physicians.[4,8]

team dynamics, and, ultimately, patient safety. This environment must be free from behaviors such as belittling or humiliation of subordinates, sarcasm, exclusion from communication, offensive or sexist remarks or threats, and hostile environments of learning.[5,6]

To create a professional environment, organizations can lead by example and establish formal policies, procedures, incentives, and informal rules for leaders. Organizations should support professional behaviors through providing protected time for training evaluations, performance feedback, and quality improvement activities. It is also recommended to provide protected on-site time away from patients so that physicians and other staff can learn about and engage in desired behaviors.[5]

IMPACT OF TRAINING ENVIRONMENT ON RESIDENTS' PROFESSIONAL DEVELOPMENT

An unprofessional training environment in an organization has a negative effect on residents and patients. Mistreatment and unethical behavior on the wards creates an environment that decreases satisfaction and fosters the depersonalization of health care professionals, which is shown to negatively impact patient care. The qualities of respect, honesty, compassion, and self-sacrifice are all compromised in this environment. Pessimism is frequently the result of mistreatment, and the published literature has taken notice of this trend as well.[10] Workplace bullying is pervasive in medical training, both in the US and internationally. According to research, 69.8% of medical residents in the US have experienced mistreatment in the workplace.[11]

A closer look at the research literature reveals the self-perpetuating nature of mistreatment and abuse in the medical work environment. Senior residents prone to misconduct likely suffered similar insults in the past and are, either knowingly or unknowingly, carrying on the "tradition" of harassment. Accordingly, it is all the more disturbing that 77.3% of the reported abuses came from senior residents.[10] This implies that senior residents perpetuate the mistreatment, failing to empathize with similarly situated first-year residents or to self-correct the errors in their professional conduct. Abusive, unprofessional behavior is counter to the principles of compassion and respect, and sets a standard that discards empathy, begging the question: if physicians cannot empathize with their peers, how can they empathize with their patients?

Studies have reported that when faculty are evaluated for respectful treatment of students, complaints about mistreatment drop by half almost immediately.[12] Within the health care work environment, collegiality and cooperation is essential to teamwork and enhances patient safety. There is no dichotomy in professionalism. One cannot be ethical to patients and malicious to colleagues or co-workers. Virtues of integrity, accountability, and compassion must be more than grand concepts applied to clinical situations. Professionalism must rigorously encompass all aspects of care, even when patients are not physically present, and be a constant guide for regulating and correcting misconduct.

Elements that promote professionalism and trust among medical trainees and the health care team include communication and teamwork, conflict resolution, stress management, and the presence of a supportive community. By investing in programs that contribute to a more professional training environment, which leads to more productive and professional physicians, organizations can contribute to better patient care. It is difficult to teach compassion to patients in an environment that has no compassion for its own physicians.

MEDRAP'S APPROACH TO FACILITATING ORGANIZATIONAL PROFESSIONALISM

Ethics seminars and policies supporting the identification, prevention, and management of unprofessional behavior are useful, but are insufficient to fundamentally change behavior. One of the fundamental goals of the MedRAP program, consistent and ongoing throughout implementation, is to foster and enhance professionalism in everyday practice. It is woven throughout all program sessions. Professionalism must rigorously encompass all aspects of care—even when patients are not physically present—as a constant guide for regulating and correcting misconduct. ACGME also has requirements for residency programs that contribute to organizational professionalism and are met by MedRAP, such as:

- To create a safe environment for residents to meet monthly and be able to self-reflect and share experiences with peers and senior residents
- To empower residents to participate in organizational problem-solving to improve hospital efficiency and patient care by teaching them techniques implemented in industry

Establishing an Ongoing Foundation of Organizational Professionalism

At its onset, MedRAP establishes a positive organizational culture, advising participants in the first session that professionalism in this residency program is evaluated not only by how they treat their patients, but also by how they treat each other.

The MedRAP sessions provide a forum for residents to meet monthly with an independent facilitator, sharing confidential feedback about problems and issues they encounter in their daily work on the hospital wards. They receive honest feedback, suggestions, and support from peers, senior residents, and the facilitator on how to best handle and resolve these issues.

When necessary, the facilitator and the GLs actively assist in conflict resolution, which cultivates a supportive community that is reported to contribute to physicians' professionalism.[8] Addressing problems soon after they are reported contributes to the PGY-1's empowerment, which is associated with burnout reduction and enhanced professional behavior. For example, if a PGY-1 experiences difficulty with a team leader in the hospital wards, the facilitator and GLs can provide advice on how to handle the situation in several ways:

- Approach the team leader and clarify issues utilizing a constructive approach
- Discuss the issue diplomatically and in a non-accusatory way with the team leader
- Alert the chief resident to the situation, and request that he/she join rounds with the team, and collect more feedback

Fostering Supportive Leadership

Organizations should choose leaders and mentors that best foster and sustain the values and behaviors of professionalism. There are common elements among leaders that are critical in promoting professional values and behaviors. Leaders and mentors should:

- Directly engage in efforts to support professional behaviors through modeling

- Participate in providing constructive feedback and supportive systems and structures
- Clearly articulate and follow the organization's values and behavioral expectations

MedRAP helps instill professionalism by identifying senior residents who are exemplary professional role models, and choosing them to be group leaders and mentors. The leadership training session for GLs emphasizes the attributes described above. Mentorship is also an important element in preventing burnout, since it helps facilitate a supportive work environment.

Meeting regularly with these GLs, selected for their professionalism and for being positive role models, helps shape the behaviors of the PGY-1 residents. The GLs often assist the PGY-1 residents with advice and with communication with their colleagues, and by providing support and advice on how to handle conflicts effectively.

Guidelines for Addressing Mistreatment

Most of the time, conflict is a result of genuine misunderstandings, preventable errors, process failures, or personal oversights, and can be resolved by clarifying miscommunications. Occasionally, however, there is unprofessional conduct involved. Residents should be asked to report when they are mistreated or when they observe senior residents or faculty exhibiting unprofessional behaviors, such as:

- Making offensive sexist or racist remarks
- Belittling or humiliating others
- Exhibiting hostility
- Using inappropriate threats

When conflict and mistreatment are severe, senior residents or faculty should be approached promptly, and unprofessional conduct should be addressed. Intervention includes facilitator communication with chief residents and/or program director, with the permission of the PGY-1 resident. GLs may address the issue with their colleagues, and solutions are devised in a collaborative manner, maintaining the PGY-1's anonymity, if possible.

Quality Improvement Sessions

In Chapter 2, we briefly introduced Quality Improvement (QI) sessions. During these sessions, confidential feedback is collected to identify systematic errors and conduct organizational problem-solving for affiliated hospitals (see Chapter 15). QI sessions also support efforts to foster professionalism within the organization.

- In the QI session, residents identify the best and most professional faculty with whom they have worked. Based on participants' feedback, the residency program can establish a special award to acknowledge the particular faculty.

- In the QI questionnaire, the residents identify faculty members exhibiting unprofessional behaviors. Residents may be concerned that departmental evaluation forms would not maintain their anonymity, potentially resulting in retribution and negatively impacting their recommendation letters.

- The information is communicated to the program management. Since it is presented towards the middle of the PGY-1 year, it is easier to maintain the reporting residents' anonymity.

Individual Assistance

Individual assistance (covered in Chapter 7) is among the ongoing components of the program that assists with facilitating professional behavior. When individual residents experience personal or professional difficulties, they may not function optimally. Effectively addressing these issues contributes to improving residents' adjustment and well-being, which is associated with professional behavior. This approach cultivates positive relationships and fosters professional behavior; the residents feel their problems are being addressed in a supportive environment, which, in turn, helps them to be more compassionate to their patients.

Addressing ACGME Milestones in Promoting Physician Professionalism

In addition to the ongoing organizational mechanisms that are in place to promote organizational professionalism that impacts the young physicians' individual professional development, the program has numerous activities that are designed to develop individual professional behaviors, such as understanding cultural diversity, dealing with personal biases, and handling moral dilemmas. These follow the ACGME recommendations for professionalism milestones and will be discussed in detail in the topic sessions.

ACGME PROFESSIONALISM MILESTONES ADDRESSED BY MEDRAP

TABLE I: ACGME PROFESSIONALISM MILESTONES

CHAPTER/SESSION	MILESTONES ADDRESSED
Chapter 9 Developing Customized Orientations	• Follow formal policies (PA2) • Maintain ethical relationships with industry (PE2) • Recognize and manage subtler conflicts of interest (PE3) • Dress and behave appropriately (PF1) • Ensure prompt completion of clinical, administrative and curricular tasks (PF3)
Chapter 10 Building Time Management Skills	• Document and report clinical information truthfully (PA1) • Accept personal errors and honestly acknowledge them (PA3) • Respond promptly and appropriately to clinical responsibilities including but not limited to calls and pages (PD1) • Ensure prompt completion of clinical, administrative and curricular tasks (PF3) • Recognize and address personal, psychological, and physical limitations that may affect professional performance (PF4) • Recognize the need to assist colleagues in the provision of duties (PF7)
Chapter 11 Discussing Code Status	• Demonstrate empathy and compassion to all patients (PB1) • Demonstrate a commitment to relieve pain and suffering (PB2) • Provide support (physical, psychological, social and spiritual) for dying patients and their families (PB3) • Recognize when it is necessary to advocate for individual patient needs (PG1) • Effectively advocate for individual patient needs (PG2)

Chapter 12
Interacting with Patients' Families

- Demonstrate empathy and compassion to all patients (PB1)
- Carry out timely interactions with colleagues, patients, and their designated caregivers (PD2)
- Recognize and manage obvious conflicts of interest, such as caring for family members and professional associates as patients (PE1)
- Maintain appropriate professional relationships with patients, families and staff (PF2)
- Recognize when it is necessary to advocate for individual patient needs (PG1)
- Effectively advocate for individual patient needs (PG2)

Chapter 13
Improving Patient-Physician Relationship

- Carry out timely interactions with colleagues, patients, and their designated caregivers (PD2)
- Recognize and manage obvious conflicts of interest, such as caring for family members and professional associates as patients (PE1)
- Maintain appropriate professional relationships with patients, families and staff (PF2)
- Recognize and address personal, psychological, and physical limitations that may affect professional performance (PF4
- Recognize when it is necessary to advocate for individual patient needs (PG1)
- Effectively advocate for individual patient needs (PG2)

Chapter 14
Breaking Bad News

- Demonstrate empathy and compassion to all patients (PB1)
- Demonstrate a commitment to relieve pain and suffering (PB2)
- Provide support (physical, psychological, social and spiritual) for dying patients and their families (PB3)
- Recognize when it is necessary to advocate for individual patient needs (PG1)
- Effectively advocate for individual patient needs (PG2)

Chapter 15
Cultivating Systems-Based Practice Skills

- Follow formal policies (P-A2)
- Communicate constructive feedback to other members of the health care team (P-C1)
- Carry out timely interactions with colleagues, patients, and their designated caregivers (P-D2)
- Recognize and manage subtler conflicts of interest (P-E3)
- Maintain appropriate professional relationships with patients, families and staff (P-F2)
- Ensure prompt completion of clinical, administrative and curricular tasks (P-F3)
- Serve as a professional role model for more junior colleagues (e.g. medical students, interns) (P-F6)
- Recognize the need to assist colleagues in the provision of duties (P-F7)
- Recognize when it is necessary to advocate for individual patient needs (P-G1)
- Effectively advocate for individual patient needs (P-G2)

Chapter 16
Developing Emotionally Intelligent Leaders

- Communicate constructive feedback to other members of the health care team (PC1)
- Recognize, respond to and report impairment in colleagues or substandard care via peer review process (PC2)
- Recognize the scope of his/her abilities and ask for supervision and assistance appropriately (PF5)
- Serve as a professional role model for more junior colleagues (e.g. medical students, interns) (PF6)
- Recognize the need to assist colleagues in the provision of duties (PF7)

Chapter 17
Strategies for Effective Team Management

- Provide leadership for a team that respects patient dignity and autonomy (PB4)
- Communicate constructive feedback to other members of the health care team (PC1)
- Recognize, respond to and report impairment in colleagues or substandard care via peer review process (PC2)
- Recognize the scope of his/her abilities and ask for supervision and assistance appropriately (PF5)
- Serve as a professional role model for more junior colleagues (e.g. medical students, residents) (PF6)
- Recognize the need to assist colleagues in the provision of duties (PF7)

SECTION 4

SESSION TOPICS

The MedRAP program is designed to address real, rather than assumed needs. After the extensive needs analysis, session topics are determined in order to meet the evolving needs of incoming residents and facilitate the transition from medical school to residency. The following chapters discuss session structure for selected topics, selection rationale, and specific facilitator tips.

The main goal and objectives for each chapter provide a pathway for implementation. The strategies and guidelines on how to design a session are based on the cumulative collective wisdom of the group leaders regarding ways to address specific challenges, as well as selected approaches collected by the facilitator from a wide range of leading researchers in different disciplines.

SESSION TOPICS AT-A-GLANCE

Chapter 9 June	**Developing Customized Orientations**	**Organizational Skills**
Chapter 10 July	**Building Time Management Skills**	**Organizational Skills**
Chapter 11 August	**Discussing Code Status**	**Communication Skills**
Chapter 12 September	**Interacting with Patients' Families**	**Communication Skills**
Chapter 13 October	**Improving Patient-Physician Relationship**	**Communication Skills**
Chapter 14 November	**Breaking Bad News**	**Communication Skills**
Chapter 15 December - March	**Cultivating Systems-Based Practice Skills**	**Quality Improvement/ Management Skills**
Chapter 16 April	**Developing Emotionally Intelligent Leaders**	**Leadership Skills**
Chapter 17 May	**Strategies for Effective Team Management**	**Leadership Skills**

CHAPTER 9:

DEVELOPING CUSTOMIZED ORIENTATIONS

The first MedRAP session is dedicated to program orientation. Facilitating the transition of new health care professionals into an organization can be challenging; some associated challenges are described below.

Turnover

Many organizations experience turnover when employees move on to other jobs and new employees replace them. These transitions usually occur throughout the year, typically affecting a relatively small number of employees. "Cohort turnover" is defined as the exit of many workers, at a single point in time, coupled with a similarly large influx of new workers. Teaching hospitals experience an annual "cohort turnover" that impacts more than 100,000 house staff in the United States and can lead to: [1]

- Decreased productivity due to disruption in operations
- Loss of tacit knowledge held by departing, more experienced physicians
- Decrease in the number of physicians familiar with the clinical system
- Decline in the clinical experience of physicians in the system
- Drop in the cumulative experience of the teaching hospital's workforce, as many of the senior residents graduate and depart, leaving new residents responsible for patient care

Implications of Cohort Turnover for Patient Care

Changeovers in care teams, particularly those that result from trainee switches, raise critical questions for patients, health care systems, and training programs. A body of research has been produced as a result of interest in the impact on patient care during this large changeover.[2-5]

Mortality and inefficiency of care has been reported by some studies to increase at the end of the academic year, when new residents begin their training at the same time that many senior residents graduate.[1] At the onset of internship, many PGY-1 residents experience high levels of anxiety and a lack of confidence in many job-related tasks. An increased incidence of hospital errors has been reported when junior doctors commence work at a new hospital.[6] Research suggests that poor outcomes related to patient care among PGY-1 residents, regardless of their previous clinical experience, are greater at the beginning of the academic year.[6] Factors that can impact their performance include: familiarity with the working environment, teamwork, and communication with other health care team members. In fact, cohort turnover of residents has been such a widespread phenomenon that it has been termed the "July effect" or "July phenomenon" in the United States and the "August killing season" in the United Kingdom.[1] This time is often considered to be the worst time of the year to be admitted to the hospital. Although there has been some controversy regarding the true prevalence of this issue,[7] multiple studies have suggested this phenomenon exists and that program directors believe it exists. Thus, implementing programs to mitigate this phenomenon is desirable from an institutional point of view. To mitigate potential care deficiencies in July, residency programs have implemented various changes. Further evaluation is necessary to determine the efficacy of these interventions on trainee education and patient safety.[8-11]

Rotation Changes

In many respects, physicians' adaptation process to new clinical and nonclinical responsibilities is an ongoing process, continuing as long as the individual is a resident. However, a great deal of the process tends to be compressed into a relatively short period of time. While the first few weeks of PGY-1 training are most important for adjustment, the entire first year of residency is a time of transition, as residents switch rotations frequently. The quality of orientations to new rotations varies, depending on the skills of the senior resident team leader or the attending physician in private hospitals.

Managing Residents' Expectations

New entrants to the helping professions frequently exhibit an unusually high degree of motivation and desire to help other people. When they are unable to have the expected positive impact on other people's lives, frustration and subsequent burnout frequently follow. Many new residents enter residency with unrealistic expectations and goals about their role as young physicians, based on what is frequently an incomplete or incorrect perception of their new role, which increases the likelihood that they are going to experience dissatisfaction, stress, and burnout.[12]

BENEFITS OF WELL-DESIGNED ORIENTATIONS

Effective orientation to health care organizations is crucial for junior doctors making the transition from medical school to residency. Comprehensive, well thought-out training can reduce adjustment periods for residents, accelerate the learning curve regarding activities related to patient care, and establish a solid foundation for their performance. Effective transitions of PGY-1 residents can reduce the negative impact of the July effect. Residency programs can help by designing effective orientations, time management training, and priority-setting activities to accelerate the learning curve prior to residency.[13]

Orientation of new junior medical staff to an unfamiliar hospital work environment is an important task; however, it can also be time consuming and repetitive.[14] For doctors, the early postgraduate years are a compelling and challenging time. PGY-1 residents must adjust to change as they rotate through different clinical units every several weeks, while at the same time maintaining a high standard of patient care. This makes a relevant and effective orientation process, together with effective patient handover, critically important. Effective orientation reduces new residents' anxiety, allowing them to rapidly become qualified members of the health care team.

While hospitals need to address certain mandatory obligations during the orientation process, programs consisting of long didactic lectures have not been found to be beneficial to new residents' needs. More lecture time does not necessarily equate to greater knowledge retention. Lecture style orientations are often considered dull and boring, with too much information imparted in too little time. Well-structured, resident-focused orientation is vital, and the orientation process ideally continues for some months during the internship year.[14]

Formal orientation programs that encompass clinical, clerical and procedural skills have been demonstrated to increase competency and confidence in junior doctors. To minimize the problems associated with the July effect, the development of formal orientation programs in residency is critical. Additionally, orientation helps PGY-1s set realistic expectations for working inside their particular organization.

New residents come to residency training programs from different medical schools all over the country, and often they do not possess the same level of skills and are unfamiliar with navigating the system. Accelerating and structuring the informal training and facilitating the transfer of knowledge from senior residents to the incoming residents to help them function effectively is especially important to ensure quality of care.

WHY DO RESIDENTS NEED ORIENTATION?	TO HELP ORIENT RESIDENTS, PROGRAMS SHOULD:
• To ease the transition from medical school to the clinical setting	• Design orientation sessions carefully based on a needs analysis
• To gain a realistic idea of what is expected of them, clarify their role, and to relieve concerns	• Impart a realistic idea of what the job is going to look like
• To become familiar with the work environment and the bureaucratic system associated with each hospital	• Clearly delineate expectations and relieve concerns
• To learn new tasks, best practices, and develop essential skills	• Offer tips and tools that will help them function more effectively in each hospital system
• To facilitate the integration of theory and practice	• Create formal mechanisms for resident support
• To learn new responsibilities in the hospital work environment	• Consolidate and disseminate existing knowledge, attitudes, and skills that are not part of formal training

MEDRAP'S APPROACH TO ORIENTATION

To accelerate the PGY-1 transition, the MedRAP approach utilizes several techniques, anticipating problems residents are likely to encounter in the hospital and training environment, and providing information to help them function more effectively. In order to create an effective orientation, a thorough needs analysis asks senior residents to evaluate their own orientation experience. The information is collected through written and oral feedback, and is analyzed and categorized with the assistance of senior residents who have already made the transition and developed strategies to function effectively. The most helpful strategies and practices are selected, and handouts are created for the new PGY-1 residents.

In the MedRAP orientation, senior residents are asked to reflect on their orientation to the residency and to respond to these questions:

- What they found helpful or not helpful
- What were their most important concerns
- What expectations did they have that were not met
- What do they know now that they did not know back then (information that would help the PGY-1 residents)
- What helpful information were they not told about the residency program or the different affiliated hospitals

The senior residents' comments included the following points:

- Orientation is frequently perceived as inadequate, conducted in a lecture style with too much information they could not assimilate.

- The written orientation material they got was often out of date.
- They would have appreciated meeting with their peers and senior residents in small groups where they could be active and ask questions.
- Meeting senior residents and peers in a relaxed environment is an important part of the orientation.
- Written, succinct orientation packages should be provided before residents start new rotation.
- Packages should be developed and updated with active involvement of the residents.
- They would have benefited from practical, realistic, problem-focused discussion.

Following the recommendations, MedRAP's first meeting is conducted at the end of the departmental orientation. Residents are divided into their pre-determined peer groups (10-12 PGY-1 residents) and meet with the senior resident GLs assigned to their group. Small groups encourage the residents to get to know each other better and begin to create a supportive community, which is important to their well-being.

It is important to give residents a realistic picture of the job they are about to undertake and set realistic expectations, as having unrealistic and unmet expectations is correlated with burnout.[15] Since there is variability in team leaders' orientations in hospital wards, having handouts helps streamline orientations to different services, and providing these tips can help the incoming residents later.

MEDRAP ORIENTATION SESSION GOALS AND OBJECTIVES

MAIN GOAL:

To help facilitate an effective and efficient transition for PGY-1 residents from medical school to residency.

OBJECTIVES:

- ◉ To help set realistic expectations for the residency experience

- ◉ To provide residents with organizational tips, strategies, and tools that will help them function more effectively

- ◉ To alleviate pre-identified typical concerns PGY-1 residents have when entering the new hospital systems

- ◉ To create a supportive and safe environment in which the residents can ask honest questions and cultivate relationships with peers and mentors

Residents also have concerns regarding specific issues that are easier to address in small groups, such as: their roles in CPR (cardiopulmonary resuscitation); pronouncing death; who they can turn to for help in rotations without a senior resident; where they can get help when they need to conduct medical procedures they are not comfortable performing.

MEDRAP'S ORIENTATION AGENDA

The MedRAP groups meet simultaneously at the end of each departmental orientation. The facilitator does not attend small group meetings, but is in the vicinity for assistance. The orientation meeting is carefully designed during the group leaders' preparation meeting. Each group leader is assigned a task, the third-year

A TYPICAL SMALL GROUP ORIENTATION AGENDA

I.   Introduction of Group Leaders
II. Introduction of Group Members
III. Typical discussion points
   - You should NEVER feel alone - asking for help is your job! You are never alone in a code.
   - Hierarchy of support (follow until you get an adequate response): co-PGY-1s, upper level resident, other upper level residents (ER/units), Chief Residents, attending physician, program director
   - Don't be afraid to call rapid response or code
   - Discussion of "The Art of Floating," created to help incoming residents during float call, which highlights important points, such as:
     ○ Strengths and weaknesses of the particular hospital system
     ○ Different bureaucratic procedures
     ○ Utilizing computer systems
     ○ How the intensive care units operate in the particular hospital
     ○ Tips for working with the emergency room in the hospital
   - "Tips for Incoming Residents" packet: created to highlight important points for the first few days of residency for the individual affiliated hospitals
IV. Discussion of "Death Pronouncement" card - since death pronouncement is typically a cause for anxiety among incoming residents, a card outlining best practices was created, suitable for residents to carry in their lab coats.
V.   Questions
VI. Exchange of contact information

group leader usually leads the meeting, and the meeting agenda is pre-determined and identical in all groups.

The orientation packet and presentation include information to help the PGY-1 residents work efficiently within each hospital. It includes advice from senior residents, information about beginning a rotation at each of the three different hospitals, and "day in the life of a PGY-1" schedules for each hospital. This information is highly customized according to specific situations and problems encountered by senior residents. For example, if residents reported that the computer orientation at one of the hospitals was deficient, a handout could be developed. The handout could provide important computer tips to accelerate the resident's daily work and thus improve care.

CREATING A CUSTOMIZED ORIENTATION

INFORMATION TO INCLUDE IN ORIENTATION:

- General logistical information specific for each hospital (such as where to get an ID badge, parking, cafeteria hours)
- Types of technology to be used
- Specific information about operations of specialized units such as Intensive Care and ER
- Strength and weakness of ancillary support
- Tips to accelerate care
- Check-in and check-out procedures
- Typical daily schedules for specific rotations and hospitals
- Conferences
- Please note: annually updated orientation materials are vital to the effective performance of the new residents

PRESENT REQUIREMENTS*: ACGME COMPETENCIES ADDRESSED BY MEDRAP ORIENTATION

Milestones Linked to Interpersonal and Communications Skills:

- Provide timely and comprehensive verbal and written communication to patients/advocates (ICS-A1)

- Effectively use verbal and nonverbal skills to create rapport with patients/families (ICS-A2)

- Use communication skills to build a therapeutic relationship (ICS-A3)

- Engage patients/advocates in shared decision-making for uncomplicated diagnostic and therapeutic scenarios (ICS-A4)

- Utilize patient centered educational strategies (ICS-A5)

- Engage patient/advocates in shared decision-making for difficult, ambiguous, or controversial scenarios (ICS-A6)

- Appropriately counsel patients about the risks and benefits of tests and procedures, highlighting cost awareness and resource allocation (ICS-A7)-

- Role model effective communication skills in challenging situations (ICS-A8)

- Effectively use an interpreter to engage patient in the clinical setting, including patient education (ICS-B1)

- Demonstrate sensitivity to differences in patients including but not limited to race, culture, gender, sexual orientation, socioeconomic status, literacy, and religious beliefs (ICS-B2)

- Actively seek to understand patient differences and views and reflects this in respectful communication and shared decision-making with the patient and the health care team (ICS-B3)

- Effectively communicate with other caregivers in order to maintain appropriate continuity during transitions of care (ICS-C1)

- Role model and teach effective communication with next caregivers during transitions of care (ICS-C2)

- Deliver appropriate, succinct, hypothesis-driven oral presentations (ICS-D1)

- Effectively communicate plan of care to all members of the health care team (ICS-D2)

- Engage in collaborative communication with all members of the health care team (ICS-D3)

---

*Milestones Linked to Core Competencies. (n.d.). Copied directly from Alliance for Academic Internal Medicine website: http://www.im.org/p/cm/ld/fid=561

- Request consultative services in an effective manner (ICS-E1)
- Clearly communicate the role of consultant to the patient, in support of the primary care relationship (ICS-E2)
- Communicate consultative recommendations to the referring team in an effective manner (ICS-E3)
- Provide legible, accurate, complete, and timely written communication that is congruent with medical standards (ICS-F1)
- Ensure succinct, relevant and patient-specific written communication (ICS-F2)

Milestones Linked to Professionalism:
- Document and report clinical information truthfully (P-A1)
- Follow formal policies (P-A2)
- Respond promptly and appropriately to clinical responsibilities including but not limited to calls and pages (P-D1)
- Carry out timely interactions with colleagues, patients, and their designated caregivers (P-D2)
- Maintain appropriate professional relationships with patients, families and staff (P-F2)
- Ensure prompt completion of clinical, administrative and curricular tasks (P-F3)
- Recognize and address personal, psychological, and physical limitations that may affect professional performance (P-F4)
- Recognize the scope of his/her abilities and ask for supervision and assistance appropriately (P-F5)
- Serve as a professional role model for more junior colleagues (e.g. medical students, interns) (P-F6)
- Recognize the need to assist colleagues in the provision of duties (P-F7)

Milestones Linked to Systems-Based Practice:
- Understand unique roles and services provided by local health care delivery systems (SBP-A1)
- Manage and coordinate care and care transitions across multiple delivery systems, including ambulatory, subacute, acute, rehabilitation and skilled nursing (SBP-A2)
- Appreciate roles of a variety of health care providers, including but not limited to consultants, therapists, nurses, home care workers, pharmacists, and social workers (SBP-B1)
- Recognize health system forces that increase the risk for error including barriers to optimal care (SBP-C1)

Milestones Linked to Practice-Based Learning and Improvement:

- Access medical information resources to answer clinical questions and support decision making (PBLI-C1)
- Maintain awareness of the situation in the moment, and respond to meet situational needs (PBLI-G1)

Milestones Linked to Patient Care:

- Recognize situations with a need for urgent or emergent medical care, including life-threatening conditions (PC-F1)
- Recognize when to seek additional guidance (PC-F2)

CHAPTER 10:

BUILDING TIME AND PATIENT CARE MANAGEMENT SKILLS

Time management and efficiency have been identified as necessary for residents to make an effective transition from medical school to residency. Yet residents often struggle to be efficient in the face of conflicting demands, difficult systematic problems, and time constraints. Operational efficiency – the ability to prioritize, to anticipate problems, and to take action in order to accomplish tasks – is a coping mechanism that greatly helps residents succeed in the training experience and has a direct impact on patient care.[1] It is possible for anyone to learn time management skills and to maximize time and productivity because it is a learned behavior.

BALANCING MULTIPLE TIME MANAGEMENT ISSUES

Competing Demands

In addition to clinical duties, residents have to manage educational responsibilities, prepare presentations about patients, and meet expectations of senior residents and senior physicians on rounds. Once the new resident enters the hospital work environment, a complex and often difficult adaptation period begins. He needs to acquire the abilities, skills, expected behaviors, and social knowledge that will help him in becoming an effective physician.

Residents are constantly shifting priorities and managing competing demands. The time management skill sets of medical students are different from those of residents, who need to constantly adapt and develop new skills to balance their professional responsibilities. The daily schedule of residents in large academic hospitals depends mostly on their year in the program, the hospital, and their specific rotations. It includes a mix of patient care and formal didactics. Patient care involves both the work required when patients are admitted to the hospital, and ongoing care of patients to whom they are assigned.

Transfer of Responsibilities

Signing out is the formal transfer of responsibility for patients between teams, and marks the beginning and end of each work day. Getting a certain set of tasks done before "sign out" is an important time management task. Learning to sign out appropriately is an essential skill that can greatly impact patient care because residents use this time to communicate patient care information. It is important to standardize sign out duties (or "handoffs") to reduce the likelihood of non- or miscommunication of patient data. Because of work hour restrictions, today's residents must leave the hospital at a certain time, and are thus faced with the challenge of determining which work to hand over and how to communicate it. Time management training aims to help residents develop effective systems for checkout.[2]

Benefits of Efficient Time Management

Time management—the process of managing time effectively, organizing, and planning how much time is spent on specific activities—plays an important role for employees in any organization, and is especially important to professionals with demanding careers. For those working in a fast-paced environment, acquiring skills in time management, learning to prioritize tasks, and keeping track of to-do lists can significantly reduce stress. Less stress impacts both professional and personal life and leads to a better work experience. Training programs in time management include both skills improvement and knowledge acquisition. Effective time management includes improving skills in:

- Prioritizing activities according to their importance
- Spending the right amount of time on activities
- Knowing how to delegate responsibilities
- Knowing the difference between important and urgent work
- Increasing allocation of time for high priority activities

THE EFFICIENT RESIDENT HAS A BETTER ABILITY TO:

- Manage time
- Anticipate problems
- Prioritize responsibilities
- Respond to urgent situations
- Simultaneously deal with multiple issues related to patient care

Improving time management skills enables young physicians to be more efficient in attending to patients' clinical care needs. In some cases, saving a life depends on knowing how to prioritize and do things quickly.

Residents have reported that time management skills acquired in medical school are helpful, but insufficient for addressing the specific challenges in the first year of residency, including supervising students, interacting with the health care team, and managing a larger number of patients. They need to develop new skills and techniques to function effectively in the hospital work environment. In addition to practical information about how to complete a task, they also need instruction in developing systems to maximize efficiency and flexibility, in case they are pulled away or have an emergency in the middle of performing a task.

MEDRAP'S APPROACH TO TIME MANAGEMENT

MedRAP's Time Management session pre-identifies important time management tips from senior residents, selects the most helpful best practices, and presents incoming PGY-1 residents with tools and handouts to accelerate their transition and improve patient care. The tools and handouts are discussed during the structured session. This session formalizes the informal training by providing information from selected senior residents. These mentors use a structured format to share their best practices and teach new PGY-1s how to manage their time efficiently.

TIME MANAGEMENT SESSION GOALS AND OBJECTIVES

MAIN GOAL:

To help residents manage their time effectively in the hospital work environment and to facilitate the transfer of important information from senior residents to PGY-1s regarding patient management.

OBJECTIVES:

- To provide general tips and best practices tips on how to manage time effectively

- To analyze their daily activities and goals in terms of time consumed

- To establish priorities for the important activities related to patient care that must be performed in the time available

- To identify methods and procedures that can accelerate clinical care by effectively utilizing ancillary services

- To help residents increase the amount of time available to attend to high priority activities

- To anticipate situations where medical mistakes are more likely to happen

- To help residents write effective notes on daily rounds and while on call

- To help residents conduct efficient "sign-outs"

GENERAL TIPS AND TOOLS TO HELP IMPROVE RESIDENTS' TIME MANAGEMENT[1,3,4]

- Be productive: there is a difference between productivity and activity; productivity has to do with identifying and doing the most important tasks to move goals forward. Many residents can be busy and active the whole day but have little accomplished.

- In order to be productive, residents have to make crucial decisions about prioritizing tasks and achieving goals.

- Learn from others: see what time management systems efficient senior residents and peers are using, and find what works best.

- Clarify expectations: make sure you understand what your seniors expect of you.

- Take action: the most successful people are proactive. Once the most important, highest yield tasks are identified, begin right away; starting a task is often the most difficult part because it requires overcoming inertia.

- Utilize medical students effectively; they learn while assisting you.

- Plan ahead: proper planning prevents poor performance, especially in public hospitals where there is variability in the efficiency of ancillary services. For example, if you need to have blood results for the purpose of ordering another test, make sure it is done early when phlebotomists usually draw blood. Contact social workers early if patient needs placement after discharge.

- Ask for help or advice with each assigned task, especially when done the first time.

- Focus on finishing tasks: to the best of your ability and unless there are emergencies, once you start a task, discipline yourself to focus until that task is complete. Unfinished tasks can be a source of distraction.

- If you can do or delegate a task in a few minutes, just do it. Completing it allows you to focus on other more important tasks at hand.

- When an unfinished task comes to mind, immediately add it to your running to do list. Regularly review the list to remove completed tasks.

- Avoid wasting time and mental energy by handling each task once. Completing a task such as finishing a chart is more efficient when it is fresh in your mind.

- Keeping multiple lists is useful: 1) in the hospital, 2) at home, 3) at the computer, etc. Clearing your mind can allow you to focus on your most important tasks.

- Aim for work-life balance: the resident lifestyle is intense. In addition to practicing time management at work, it is important to prioritize personal time.

DISCUSSION OF TYPICAL RESIDENT SCHEDULE

To develop time management skills, one useful activity is to review a typical daily schedule at a specific hospital or rotation, discussing important details to help increase the PGY-1 resident's efficiency. GLs divide into groups per hospital/rotation, and PGY-1s join the group for their current or future hospital rotation.

Once in groups, GLs lead a discussion using the "Life as a Medicine Resident" handout and review important points regarding a typical daily schedule. These small group discussions help some PGY-1 residents to feel more comfortable asking questions or providing feedback about their rotations.

Daily schedule organizational tips are provided for the following activities:

- Residents' pre-rounds
- How to handle emergencies such as "crashing patients"
- How to prioritize
- Conferences
- How to be efficient with ward work
- Writing notes
- Hospital-specific forms for tests/orders
- New admissions
- Tips for ward call
- To-do list for checkout
- Tips for discharge

MINIMIZING MEDICAL MISTAKES

New PGY-1 residents, overwhelmed with their new clinical responsibilities and unfamiliar with effective time management techniques, are more prone to making medical mistakes.[5,6] Research suggests that medical errors should rank as the third leading cause of death in the United States;[7] thus, MedRAP's time management session is focused on reducing the risk of medical mistakes. The time management session also includes a discussion of a handout, prepared and revised at the group leaders meeting. Topics include specific medications and hospital situations associated with higher risk of mistakes. This information varies by rotation or hospital and these differences are discussed. Senior residents often share their own mistakes to help the PGY-1 residents avoid making the same errors.

WRITING EFFICIENT NOTES

PGY-1 residents' notes on patients are different from medical students' notes, which are much longer. Some new residents spend a lot of time writing notes, and for effective time management it is important to instruct them in writing efficient notes. This session includes examples of good and bad notes, along with an explanation of the differences between them.

PGY-1 residents learn what to cover in their notes, focusing on pertinent and essential information. They are reminded to think about the resident on call and include important information, such as code status and contact information, while omitting unnecessary details.

PRESENT REQUIREMENTS: ACGME COMPETENCIES ADDRESSED IN TIME AND PATIENT CARE MANAGEMENT

Milestones Linked to Interpersonal and Communications Skills:

- Provide timely and comprehensive verbal and written communication to patients/advocates (ICS-A1)
- Effectively use verbal and nonverbal skills to create rapport with patients/families (ICS-A2)
- Use communication skills to build a therapeutic relationship (ICS-A3)
- Engage patients/advocates in shared decision-making for uncomplicated diagnostic and therapeutic scenarios (ICS-A4)
- Utilize patient centered educational strategies (ICS-A5)
- Engage patient/advocates in shared decision-making for difficult, ambiguous, or controversial scenarios (ICS-A6)
- Appropriately counsel patients about the risks and benefits of tests and procedures, highlighting cost awareness and resource allocation (ICS-A7)
- Role model effective communication skills in challenging situations (ICS-A8)
- Effectively use an interpreter to engage patient in the clinical setting, including patient education (ICS-B1)
- Demonstrate sensitivity to differences in patients including but not limited to race, culture, gender, sexual orientation, socioeconomic status, literacy, and religious beliefs (ICS-B2)
- Actively seek to understand patient differences and views and reflects this in respectful communication and shared decision-making with the patient and the health care team (ICS-B3)
- Effectively communicate with other caregivers in order to maintain appropriate continuity during transitions of care (ICS-C1)
- Role model and teach effective communication with next caregivers during transitions of care (ICS-C2)
- Deliver appropriate, succinct, hypothesis-driven oral presentations (ICS-D1)
- Effectively communicate plan of care to all members of the health care team (ICS-D2)
- Engage in collaborative communication with all members of the health care team (ICS-D3)
- Request consultative services in an effective manner (ICS-E1)
- Clearly communicate the role of consultant to the patient, in support of the primary care relationship (ICS-E2)

- Communicate consultative recommendations to the referring team in an effective manner (ICS-E3)
- Provide legible, accurate, complete, and timely written communication that is congruent with medical standards (ICS-F1)
- Ensure succinct, relevant and patient-specific written communication (ICS-F2)

Milestones Linked to Professionalism:
- Document and report clinical information truthfully (P-A1)
- Follow formal policies (P-A2)
- Accept personal errors and honestly acknowledge them (P-A3)
- Carry out timely interactions with colleagues, patients, and their designated caregivers (P-D2)
- Maintain ethical relationships with industry (P-E2)
- Maintain appropriate professional relationships with patients, families and staff (P-F2)
- Ensure prompt completion of clinical, administrative and curricular tasks (P-F3)
- Recognize and address personal, psychological, and physical limitations that may affect professional performance (P-F4)
- Recognize the scope of his/her abilities and ask for supervision and assistance appropriately (P-F5)
- Recognize the need to assist colleagues in the provision of duties (P-F7)

Milestones Linked to Systems-Based Practice:
- Understand unique roles and services provided by local health care delivery systems (SBP-A1)
- Manage and coordinate care and care transitions across multiple delivery systems, including ambulatory, subacute, acute, rehabilitation and skilled nursing (SBP-A2)
- Appreciate roles of a variety of health care providers, including but not limited to consultants, therapists, nursed, home care workers, pharmacists, and social workers (SBP-B1)
- Work effectively as a member within the interprofessional team to ensure safe patient care (SBP-B2)
- Recognize health system forces that increase the risk for error including barriers to optimal care (SBP-C1)
- Identify, reflect on, and learn from critical incidents such as near misses and preventable medical errors (SBP-C2)

- Dialogue with care team members to identify risk for and prevention of medical error (SBP-C3)

Milestones Linked to Practice-Based Learning and Improvement:

- Access medical information resources to answer clinical questions and support decision making (PBLI-C1)

- Effectively and efficiently search NLM databases for original clinical research articles (PBLI-C2)

- Effectively and efficiently search evidence-based summary medical information resources (PBLI-C3)

- Appraise the quality of medical information resources and select among them based on the characteristics of the clinical question (PBLI-C4)

- Respond welcomingly and productively to feedback from all members of the health care team including faculty, peer residents, students, nurses, allied health workers, patients and their advocates (PBLI-F1)

- Actively seek feedback from all members of the health care team (PBLI-F2)

- Calibrate self-assessment with feedback and other external data (PBLI-F3)

- Reflect on feedback in developing plans for improvement (PBLI-F4)

- Maintain awareness of the situation in the moment, and respond to meet situational needs (PBLI-G1)

- Reflect (in action) when surprised, applies new insights to future clinical scenarios, and reflects (on action) back on the process (PBLI-G2)

- Actively participate in teaching conferences (PBLI-H1)

- Integrate teaching, feedback and evaluation with supervision of PGY-1s' and students' patient care (PBLI-H2)

- Take a leadership role in the education of all members of the health care team (PBLI-H3)

- Recognize that disparities exist in health care among populations and that they may impact care of the patient (P-K1)

- Embrace physicians' role in assisting the public and policy makers in understanding and addressing causes of disparity in disease and suffering (P-K2)

Milestones Linked to Patient Care:

- Seek and obtain appropriate, verified, and prioritized data from secondary sources (e.g. family, records, pharmacy) (PC-A2)

- Recognize situations with a need for urgent or emergent medical care, including life-threatening conditions (PC-F1)

- Recognize when to seek additional guidance (PC-F2)

- Initiate management and stabilize patients with emergent medical conditions (PC-F6)
- Manage patients with conditions that require intensive care (PC-F7)

CHAPTER 11:

DISCUSSING CODE STATUS

Vast progress in medical care has led to an increased life expectancy and an aging population, and therefore an increased need for effective end-of-life communication between physicians and patients or their family members. It is important to make sure that invasive medical treatments are not conducted on patients who would prefer less aggressive forms of care at the end of their lives.[1] Regrettably, health care team members often fail to initiate end-of-life discussions with patients and therefore do not document patient wishes on code status.[2] This failure can lead to patients having unwanted, aggressive, and potentially futile medical care. Multiple studies have reported that unwanted life-prolonging treatments are frequently given to patients, and that open discussions on their efficacy, goals and prognosis are often lacking.[3] Utilizing effective communication techniques to discuss treatment and palliative care could improve patient care at or near the end of life.

Even when the diagnosis is incurable, aggressive treatments are provided before prognosis and goals of care are determined. Most frequently, trials of life-sustaining treatments can last days or weeks. Other complicating factors are the inability to exactly predict the time of death, a tendency to overestimate survival, and encouragement of overtreatment.

Communication and decision-making can be challenging during this period for several reasons:

- Disease can frequently cause patients to lose decision-making capacity
- Some patients prefer not to discuss their prognosis
- Living wills and advance care plans are often not available

As a result, physicians often need to help patients or their family members make the decision to move from fighting death to acceptance that the situation is terminal, which can lead to conflicts if the communication is not handled correctly.

Code status refers to patients' preferred level of medical intervention when their heart or breathing stops.

Do not resuscitate (DNR) is a written order stating a patient's wishes to withhold cardiopulmonary resuscitation (CPR) or advanced cardiac life support (ACLS) if his/her heart or breathing stops. The DNR request is typically made by the patient or an appropriate surrogate decision maker.

A DNR order impacts only treatment requiring intubation or CPR. Patients who are DNR can continue to get chemotherapy, antibiotics, dialysis, or any other necessary treatments.

An end-of-life care discussion should occur early in a patient's hospitalization and address the wide range of concerns experienced by dying patients and their families. Physicians should make sure the patient and family clearly understand the prognosis and help them achieve important end-of-life goals. The discussion of code status with patients and their families requires sensitivity, honesty, and cultural understanding. The physician should find the right balance between presenting realistic and unrealistic expectations. Studies have shown that patients choose different resuscitation options, depending on how the question is framed and what material is presented to them.[4]

The intricacies involved in discussion of code status highlight the importance of the physician's skill in discussing the topic. And yet, the discussion of end-of-life care frequently occurs too late in the course of a patient's illness. Often, patients and their families wait to explore end-of-life care options, expecting the physician to bring up the topic and inform them about the diagnosis, prognosis, and treatment. They also often expect the physician to help them make decisions that reflect the goals of the patient and family at this time of severe stress. However, multiple studies suggest that DNR communication is poor.[5] Many physicians tend to avoid the dialogue because it is an unpleasant task for them, and they often lack the training to properly discuss the issue. This difficult discussion often occurs only when necessitated by medical urgency.

Many families report conflicts with medical staff, usually involving poor communication regarding end-of-life care. They also report that when they need to make crucial decisions such as code status, they:[6]

- Do not understand even basic information about the patient's diagnosis, prognosis, or treatment

- Receive insufficient or unclear information on their loved one's diagnosis

- Feel excluded from decision-making and, as a result, experience anxiety and depression

The same studies report that family satisfaction is correlated with:

- Physician support for family decisions about end-of-life care

- How often they are allowed to express their thoughts

- Being assured that their family member would not be abandoned, would be kept comfortable, and would not suffer

Based on research regarding communication training, physicians need instruction to develop skills related to discussing code status with patients.[7] Training that teaches physicians to use proven strategies and evidence-based methods benefits patients, families, physicians, and the medical system as a whole.

Because medical residents in large academic centers are on duty most of the time, and especially at night, they are often tasked with discussing resuscitation decisions. They are often first responders when the patient's condition deteriorates. Unfortunately, studies suggest that the quality of their discussions is poor.[8,9] Residents, as well as senior physicians, often:

- Do not provide sufficient information to allow patients to make an informed decision

- Do not clearly describe the likelihood of survival with CPR

- Convey risk and benefit using only vague expressions of probability

- Demonstrate few empathic comments

- Seldom ask about the patient's personal values to help them make more appropriate decisions

- Pursue their own agendas, based on their own personal judgment, encouraging DNR decisions instead of responding to patient concerns

Even if they have training regarding code status discussions, physicians may not perform well under the stress of environmental circumstances such as work overload, multiple clinical responsibilities, and sleep deprivation. The old assumption in medical residencies regarding communication skills was that anyone could do it after observing a more experienced physician. However, proper discussions have such an impact on patients, families, and the medical system, that communication should be taught just as any other medical skill.

Given the importance of understanding and addressing sociocultural factors in the medical encounter, cross-cultural education is also increasingly important in communication training for physicians. Due to increasing diversity in the US, the risk for misunderstandings between patients and physicians from different cultural backgrounds regarding the end of life is also increasing.[10] Cultural factors shape how individuals view end-of-life issues, such as suffering, hope and truth telling, life-prolonging technology, and decision-making styles at the end of life. Physicians need to develop cross-cultural understanding and communication techniques to increase the likelihood that both the process and the outcomes of the discussion about end-of-life care are satisfactory for patients and families. Communication and clinical decision-making can be impacted by sociocultural differences between patients and physicians. Based on their sociocultural background, patients tend to present distinct perspectives, values, and beliefs regarding health and illness. These include patients':[11]

- Variations in presentation of their symptoms
- Ability to understand prescribed management strategies
- Expectations of care
- Adherence to preventive measures and medications

Certain strategies and guidelines can help the physician achieve an effective DNR discussion, which can relieve the patient, the family, and the physician while addressing important questions regarding end-of-life care. It is important that physicians learn how to:

- Focus on the patient's concerns and goals for care
- Give patients a balanced presentation of the options that includes relevant outcome data
- Objectively present their options
- Make recommendations if needed
- Use a patient-centered approach, with open-ended questions and empathic listening

Addressing these issues in a timely and appropriate manner will help patients, families, physicians, and the health care team. If given accurate information about the low probability of survival, patients and families might choose to let go,[12] potentially saving our medical system from spending unnecessary resources to preserve a patient's life.

MEDRAP'S APPROACH TO DISCUSSION OF CODE STATUS

MedRAP's approach to helping incoming PGY-1 residents handle the issue of code status discussion focuses on the residents' needs as determined by the needs assessment feedback session. In the needs analysis, residents highlighted several important issues. They reported that while they provide much of the care to dying patients and conduct DNR discussions themselves, only a few of them received some form of training in end-of-life care. Even if they received training during medical school, it is more meaningful to receive the training during residency, when they are directly responsible to patients and their families and are actually conducting these discussions. They expressed the need for clear and practical guidelines on issues related to DNR discussions early in the year. While they observed experienced physicians discussing DNR utilizing a wide variety of approaches, the quality and effectiveness of the discussion varied. In general, residents observed inconsistency in expertise; communication skills regarding this topic did not necessarily improve with experience alone.

Based on MedRAP resident feedback, the following goals and objectives were formed for the code status discussion session:

DISCUSSION OF CODE STATUS SESSION GOALS AND OBJECTIVES

MAIN GOAL:

To provide residents with strategies, tools, and tips to help them conduct an effective code status discussion.

OBJECTIVES:

- Provide general guidelines and approaches to DNR discussions

- Provide essential factual information to better understand important variables related to code status discussions

- Provide strategies to help elicit patients' values and wishes or make recommendations when appropriate

- Identify typical difficult challenges the PGY-1 residents are likely to encounter relating to code status issues, i.e. moral dilemmas, cultural issues, and managing attending physicians who are overly optimistic about prognosis

- Facilitate self-reflection related to these difficult encounters and reactions to them

- Prepare them to deal with these challenges by identifying best practices and strategies

◉ Help residents tailor the discussions to the specific needs of patients or families

◉ Educate PGY-1 residents about prognosis after CPR and provide them with helpful statistics

◉ Provide strategies and best practices to discuss code status with different patient groups, such as:

   ○ The basically healthy patient

   ○ The patient with advanced or chronic illness

   ○ The terminally ill patient that is close to death

Due to the complexity of end-of-life discussion, the MedRAP approach to discussing code status includes both didactic and strategic components. The didactic section includes discussion of key concepts to consider for effective code status discussions. These guidelines are an important part of educating residents about discussing code status and are based on several important articles providing helpful strategies and guidelines for code status discussion.

CODE STATUS DISCUSSION DIDACTIC SECTION
Key Concepts[1,13-14]

The key concepts residents should be familiar with when discussing code status include:

Succession of responsibility:
- In the absence of an advance directive, there is a need to determine whom to communicate with about critical care decisions.
- Often, many family members are involved in these discussions, thus it is important to identify which one of them is the decision-maker.
- Since state legislation may differ in defining the hierarchy of decision-makers, it is important to refer to state law when addressing these issues.
- The most frequent hierarchy, without legal guidance, is: spouse; adult children; parents.
- Physicians should advocate for decisions that best reflect the patient's values and wishes.
- Next of kin may not be the most appropriate source for this information.

Surrogate decision-making:

- At times there will be a need to make decisions on behalf of patients without decision-making capacity.
- Lacking a formal written or oral directive expressing patient wishes for future care, surrogates are requested to provide substituted judgments, choosing what the patient would have chosen.
- If the patient's preferences are unknown, a decision should be made in the patient's best interests.
- Decision-makers are asked to put themselves in the patient's shoes to determine how the patient, if able to understand his or her condition, would make the decision.
- The family needs to understand the difference between their subjective feelings, values and judgments, and decisions that will be made with the best interest of the patient in mind.
- Family members need to be reminded that the decision may not be the same they would make for themselves; stay focused on the patient's values and wishes.
- Surrogate decision-making is often complicated by guilt that can be decreased when the family tries to approximate the patient's decisions.

Prognosis and clinical condition:

- In order to make the best decisions for the patient, the family needs to clearly understand the patient's condition and prognosis.
- Family members' expectations regarding the patient's prognosis should be assessed.
- It is important to determine, early in the discussion, the level of the family's understanding of the patient's condition and to what degree they accept the prognosis.
- Providing emotional support is very important when family members initially express concerns about the imminent death of their loved one.
- When the family cannot make a decision or provide clear direction after multiple meetings, the physician needs to have additional meetings with experts, ethics committee members and other resources.

Values directives vs. procedural directives:

- When written advance directives are not in place, other approaches can help define a patient's wishes about critical medical decisions.
- Procedural directives define which procedures or interventions should be undertaken or excluded in different situations, factoring in whether the patient is competent, or specifically expressed specific wishes regarding treatment.

- Assess the patient's values about quality of life and survival, and then attempt to identify best approaches that are consistent with those values.
- If the patient has never discussed terminal care preferences, assessing patient's values can assist in determining the patient's likely preferences. Families can be instrumental in this process.

Life-maintaining vs. supportive care:
- Families need to be assisted in determining whether their goal is maintaining the patient's comfort and dignity, or pursuing aggressive care aimed at maintaining life.
- The option of a time-limited therapeutic trial can be considered when prognosis is uncertain or family members are unable to accept the reality of the patient's approaching demise.

Legal considerations:
- State legislation regarding end-of-life decision-making should be taken into consideration when discussing end-of-life plans with a family.
- When families and physicians agree about prognosis and the patient's preferences, the courts tend to support their decisions.
- Some states require a higher burden of proof for certain substituted judgment decisions.

CODE STATUS DISCUSSION STRATEGIC SECTION
Tips, Tools, and General Guidelines[1,15-19]

Tips for advance care planning:
- Be a proactive listener
- Elicit patient's goals of care and values, and match interventions with these goals
- Use simple language
- Distinguish situations where outcomes are better, such as in the OR or during conscious sedation for procedures
- Ask about preferences in scenarios with uncertain outcomes, i.e., successful cardiac resuscitation which can result in severe anoxic brain injury
- Assess the patient's understanding of available options
- Reassess the patient's goals of care at every hospitalization

Recommended steps for discussing a DNR order:
- Establish an appropriate setting for the discussion; the earlier the better
- Explore what the patient and family understand about the illness and prognosis
- Clarify patients' expectations and goals they have for the time left

- Discuss a DNR order, including context using language patients will understand
- Respond to emotions
- Establish and implement the plan

Keep in mind that:

- Patients' preferences regarding resuscitation options are not always assessed appropriately
- DNR discussions should be addressed early enough so that patients can participate in decisions regarding resuscitation
- Physicians need to make sure to provide adequate information to allow patients to make informed decisions
- Advance directives are important tools for providing care in keeping with patients' wishes
- The popularity of advance directives has grown tremendously, despite debate about their effectiveness
- Surrogate decision making is often required for elderly patients at the end of life
- Both a living will and a durable power of attorney for health care appear to have a significant effect on the outcomes of decision making
- When completed, advance directives are often unavailable upon hospitalization and it is advisable to instruct patient to keep multiple copies and advise family members
- Hospital-based physicians often discuss code status with patients they have not previously met

Frequent misconceptions even after discussions are that:

- CPR survival is much higher than it is in reality
- Ventilated patients could talk
- Ventilators were oxygen tanks
- People on ventilators were in a coma

PRESENT REQUIREMENTS: ACGME COMPETENCIES ADDRESSED IN DISCUSSION OF CODE STATUS

Milestones Linked to Interpersonal and Communications Skills:

- Provide timely and comprehensive verbal and written communication to patients/advocates (ICS-A1)
- Effectively use verbal and nonverbal skills to create rapport with patients/families (ICS-A2)
- Use communication skills to build a therapeutic relationship (ICS-A3)
- Engage patients/advocates in shared decision-making for uncomplicated diagnostic and therapeutic scenarios (ICS-A4)
- Utilize patient centered educational strategies (ICS-A5)
- Engage patient/advocates in shared decision-making for difficult, ambiguous, or controversial scenarios (ICS-A6)
- Appropriately counsel patients about the risks and benefits of tests and procedures, highlighting cost awareness and resource allocation (ICS-A7)
- Role model effective communication skills in challenging situations (ICS-A8)
- Effectively use an interpreter to engage patient in the clinical setting, including patient education (ICS-B1)
- Demonstrate sensitivity to differences in patients including but not limited to race, culture, gender, sexual orientation, socioeconomic status, literacy, and religious beliefs (ICS-B2)
- Actively seek to understand patient differences and views and reflects this in respectful communication and shared decision-making with the patient and the health care team (ICS-B3)
- Effectively communicate with other caregivers in order to maintain appropriate continuity during transitions of care (ICS-C1)
- Role model and teach effective communication with next caregivers during transitions of care (ICS-C2)
- Deliver appropriate, succinct, hypothesis-driven oral presentations (ICS-D1)
- Effectively communicate plan of care to all members of the health care team (ICS-D2)
- Engage in collaborative communication with all members of the health care team (ICS-D3)
- Request consultative services in an effective manner (ICS-E1)
- Clearly communicate the role of consultant to the patient, in support of the primary care relationship (ICS-E2)

- Communicate consultative recommendations to the referring team in an effective manner (ICS-E3)
- Provide legible, accurate, complete, and timely written communication that is congruent with medical standards (ICS-F1)
- Ensure succinct, relevant and patient-specific written communication (ICS-F2)

Milestones Linked to Professionalism:
- Document and report clinical information truthfully (P-A1)
- Demonstrate empathy and compassion to all patients (P-B1)
- Demonstrate a commitment to relieve pain and suffering (P-B2)
- Provide support (physical, psychological, social, and spiritual) for dying patients and their families (P-B3)
- Provide leadership for a team that respects patient dignity and autonomy (P-B4)
- Carry out timely interactions with colleagues, patients, and their designated caregivers (P-D2)
- Recognize and manage obvious conflicts of interest, such as caring for family members and professional associates as patients (P-E1)
- Maintain appropriate professional relationships with patients, families, and staff (P-F2)
- Recognize and address personal, psychological, and physical limitations that may affect professional performance (P-F4)
- Recognize the scope of his/her abilities and ask for supervision and assistance appropriately (P-F5)
- Recognize the need to assist colleagues in the provision of duties (P-F7)
- Recognize when it is necessary to advocate for individual patient needs (P-G1)
- Effectively advocate for individual patient needs (P-G2)
- Recognize and take responsibility for situations where public health supersedes individual health (e.g. reportable infectious diseases) (P-H1)
- Treat patients with dignity, civility and respect, regardless of race, culture, gender, ethnicity, age, or socioeconomic status (P-I1)
- Recognize and manage conflict when patient values differ from their own (P-I2)
- Maintain patient confidentiality (P-J1)
- Educate and hold others accountable for patient confidentiality (P-J2)
- Recognize that disparities exist in health care among populations and that they may impact care of the patient (P-K1)
- Advocate for appropriate allocation of limited health care resources (P-K3)

Milestones Linked to Systems-Based Practice:

- Negotiate patient-centered care among multiple care providers (SBP-A3)
- Appreciate roles of a variety of health care providers, including but not limited to consultants, therapists, nursed, home care workers, pharmacists, and social workers (SBP-B1)
- Work effectively as a member within the inter professional team to ensure safe patient care (SBP-B2)
- Consider alternative solutions provided by other teammates (SBP-B3)
- Reflect awareness of common socio-economic barriers that impact patient care (SBP-D1)
- Understand how cost-benefit analysis is applied to patient care (i.e. via principles of screening tests and the development of clinical guidelines) (SBP-D2)
- Minimize unnecessary care, including tests, procedures, therapies and ambulatory or hospital encounters (SBP-E2)
- Demonstrate the incorporation of cost-awareness principles into standard clinical judgments and decision-making (SBP-E3)
- Demonstrate the incorporation of cost-awareness principles into complex clinical scenarios (SBP-E4)

Milestones Linked to Practice-Based Learning and Improvement:

- Independently appraise clinical guideline recommendations for bias and cost-benefit considerations (PBLI-D4)
- Determine if clinical evidence can be generalized to an individual patient (PBLI-E1)
- Customize clinical evidence for an individual patient (PBLI-E2)
- Communicate risks and benefits to alternative to patients (PBLI-E3)
- Integrate clinical evidence, clinical context, and patient preferences into decision-making (PBLI-E4)
- Actively participate in teaching conferences (PBLI-H1)

Milestones Linked to Patient Care:

- Acquire accurate and relevant history from the patient in an efficiently customized, prioritized, and hypothesis-driven fashion (PC-A1)
- Seek and obtain appropriate, verified, and prioritized data from secondary sources (e.g. family, records, pharmacy) (PC-A2)
- Obtain relevant historical subtleties that inform and prioritize both differential diagnoses and diagnostic plans, including sensitive, complicated, and detailed information that may not often be volunteered by the patient (PC-A3)

- Role model gathering subtle and reliable information from the patient for junior members of the health care team (PC-A4)

- Make appropriate clinical decisions based on the results of common diagnostic testing, including but not limited to routine blood chemistries, hematologic studies, coagulations tests, arterial blood gases, ECG, chest radiographs, pulmonary function tests, urinalysis, and other body fluids (PC-E1)

- Make appropriate clinical decisions based upon the results of more advanced diagnostic tests (PC-E2)

- Recognize situations with a need for urgent or emergent medical care, including life-threatening conditions (PC-F1)

- Recognize when to seek additional guidance (PC-F2)

- Provide appropriate preventive care and teach patient regarding self-care (PC-F3)

- Customize care in the context of the patient's preferences and overall health (PC-F10)

- Provide internal medicine consultation for patients with more complex clinical problems requiring detailed risk assessment (PC-G2)

Milestones Linked to Medical Knowledge:

- Demonstrate sufficient knowledge of socio-behavioral sciences including but not limited to health care economics, medical ethics and medical education (MK-A9)

CHAPTER 12:

INTERACTING WITH PATIENTS' FAMILIES

Health care communication is a skill that is critical to safe and effective medical practice; it can and must be taught since it influences, among other things, accurate diagnosis, patient treatment plan, improved patient knowledge, adherence to treatment regimen and outcome, and adaptation to illness.[1] Improving communication with patients and families enables more effective, efficient, and empathic care.

It is important to establish good working relationships with families and to recognize their importance to the patient's health care experience. Family caregivers play a major role in taking care of more than 30 million individuals with acute and chronic illness. Families in the US provide care for about 90% of dependent patients with acute and chronic physical illness, cognitive impairments and mental health conditions.[2] Approximately 43.5 million family caregivers over the age of 18 helped patients manage illnesses and treatment recommendations in 2015.[3] Patients depend on family caregivers for help with daily activities such as navigating the hospital system, managing complex care, and communicating with physicians and other health care team members. Patients' overall safety can improve when family members play an active role in patient care by: providing important information about the patient's condition; contributing to the patient's understanding about a medical diagnosis; ensuring compliance with treatment regimen; and preventing medical errors and inefficiencies in the health care system.[4]

Patient- and family-centered care (PFCC) is a relatively new strategic approach that is changing the way hospitals care for their patients by emphasizing staff satisfaction, decreasing costs, and improving patient outcomes. Participating hospitals endorse core values such as recognizing the important role of family members in the patients' health care experience, establishing supportive relationships with them, and empowering patients to utilize the health care system effectively. Hospitals that implement PFCC experience higher satisfaction ratings by patients, families, and staff, as well as improved patient health outcomes.[5,6]

This approach recommends that health care providers:

- Provide information in terms patients and family members can understand
- Encourage families to participate in the care of their loved ones
- Take time to understand any influences of language, health literacy, or social, educational, or cultural factors on patients or families
- Establish a respectful relationship, and incorporate patient and family preferences and values in care goals and plans
- Identify and address patient communication needs promptly, such as assistance for family members whose preferred language is not English or who have sensory or communication impairments
- Disclose and acknowledge any medical errors promptly
- Consider individual patient values along with possible language barriers, cultural issues, health literacy, and other factors

Effective communication with patients and their families is an essential tool for accurate diagnosis, development of a successful treatment plan, and compliance of patients. Empathic communication has been shown to be an essential skill that can lead to better patient and family satisfaction, improved outcomes, and also reduction in malpractice suits. Many physicians believe that if they follow established standard procedures in their practices, they will not be sued. However, differences between physicians who have and have not been sued cannot be fully explained by the quality of care they provide. In fact, studies suggest that a high percentage of medicolegal actions against physicians involve communication breakdowns between physicians, patients and families,[7-9] such as:

- Poor delivery of information
- Failure to understand patient and family perspectives
- Failure to solicit and incorporate patient's values into the plan of care
- Perceptions of desertion

Ultimately, patients and families satisfied with the communication and attention received are more likely to forgive medical mistakes. When faced with a bad outcome, patients and families are likely to reflect on whether the physicians were caring and compassionate, and whether they invested the needed time in the patient's management.

Effective health care communication is responsive to the needs of the whole patient and family dynamic; it is essential to patient-centered and family-centered care.

However, physicians, at times, have difficulties communicating with a patient's family. Many physicians avoid interaction altogether because they feel that the families are not under their direct care. Research also suggests that physicians tend to avoid patients and families when they find them difficult.[10-11] Avoiding interactions with families leaves the physician unprepared to deal with other issues related to patient care, such as early detection of a developing problem or the discovery of other vital information.

In addition to these general issues, some families are particularly difficult for many physicians to handle. These patients' families can be a great source of stress, anger, and irritation, especially for an inexperienced physician. Dysfunctional families with maladaptive dynamics,[10] as well as healthy families in stressful situations, can exhibit difficult behaviors, challenging to even experienced health care professionals. Physicians need to develop effective communication skills and strategies to effectively handle these situations. If the physician lacks an understanding of complex family dynamics and the communication techniques required, it can have an adverse impact on patient care and satisfaction. In fact, residents participating in MedRAP consistently recommended that the session regarding family interaction be offered early in the year, as this was a considerable challenge for them.

A patient's family can be difficult for physicians for a variety of reasons, such as:

- Lack of training in communicating with family members
- Feeling outnumbered by family members
- Inability to provide the type of support the family needs
- Feeling the family takes too much of their time
- Feeling the family can become another difficult variable they must deal with

If physicians can learn to recognize basic categories and characteristics of families they have difficulty managing, and acquire tools to work with them, they will be able to communicate and manage them more effectively. Communication training can help physicians navigate family dynamics and have more control over their patients' treatment as a whole.

Many medical educators are concerned about the loss of empathy in medical trainees, due, in part, to current medical education methods and role models. Health care communication is currently learned primarily through trial and error, partly due to the variability of mentors' communication skills. Several studies have demonstrated that empathy can be either eroded during medical training, or developed and taught, and also suggest that faculty in medical school could benefit from communication skills training as well.[12-14] Empathetic physicians elicit patient concerns more accurately and effectively address the needs of patients and their families. Empathy impacts quality of care and patient satisfaction and contributes to reducing cost of care.[1] Despite specific requirements and recommendations of the ACGME, empathic communication is still under-emphasized in addressing the needs of patients and families. The training emphasis on data collection and clinical care does not adequately equip medical trainees to fully meet the needs of patients and their families.

MEDRAP'S APPROACH TO COMMUNICATION WITH FAMILIES

While residents receive informal training on dealing with families as they observe senior residents in similar situations, formalized training can help residents communicate with families more effectively. Identifying challenges specific to resident experiences and providing professional strategies and best practices can improve care, save time, and reduce stress.

To teach family skills, the focus in the program is on various communication challenges. Communication can be viewed as a cognitively-based, learned intellectual process that requires the understanding of feelings. Breaking communication into components allows an enriched understanding of a person's feelings to develop, which can make communication more effective. When analyzed and broken down, even poor behavior can lead to better understanding and more productive communication.

It is possible to break down behaviors into their components and analyze why some communication patterns are more helpful than others. It is also possible to anticipate typical difficult situations that residents encounter when interacting with patients and families, so they can be prepared to handle them. For example, in the self-reflection section of the session, residents are asked to describe and analyze challenging family situations encountered by their senior residents or attending physicians. They are asked to analyze specific communication styles they observed and identify which behaviors disarmed or led to better rapport with the family, as well as behaviors that caused the situation to escalate or resulted in hostile reactions.

INTERACTING WITH PATIENTS' FAMILIES
SESSION GOALS AND OBJECTIVES

MAIN GOAL:

◉ To manage families effectively and contribute to patient care and satisfaction by meeting the following objectives:

OBJECTIVES:

◉ To employ some basic techniques of managing and communicating with families, recognizing the basic categories of challenging families to anticipate and respond to their dynamics

◉ To manage the interaction with each family category

◉ To tailor the communication to each family

◉ To set boundaries and limits in a positive way

◉ To prevent potential problems

GENERAL TIPS AND TOOLS FOR HANDLING FAMILIES[*1,4,10,15-17]

Being hospitalized is a very stressful experience for patients and their families. It leads to anxiety and stronger than usual emotional responses, and is often a set-up for disagreement and conflicts. With careful listening, compromising, and patient and family education, all parties can have a better experience during a tough time.

It is important that the physician exhibit interest, empathy, and appreciation for multiple points of view. Most importantly, residents should be taught to demonstrate an interest in the family members as people with their own needs and history. The following general guidelines can be helpful:

- **Acknowledge family's distress.** All family members are impacted by the challenges of living with a very sick family member. It is helpful to address the immediate emotional and practical needs of the patient and family members. These can include helplessness, guilt, or shame. It is also important to understand that in this stressful situation, old family conflicts can be reactivated around decision-making, and the family may need help to separate these conflicts from the immediate medical situation. The resident can facilitate communication about the illness, treatment-related issues, and necessary decisions. Serious conflict among family members, particularly related to death and dying, often makes these processes far more painful, and stunts family growth for years to come.

- **Apply systematic thinking when interacting with families**. Residents encounter different kinds of families over the years of their training. Many learn about different types of families and develop communication styles suited to each one. However, they need an opportunity to reflect, analyze their experiences, and learn to categorize families they encounter, supplemented with techniques that can assist them to systematically approach each unique situation.

- **Think "family categories."** Families can be divided into broad basic categories. These categories can overlap, and families can have characteristics of more than one category. If residents learn to see patterns and can be trained to employ strategies that work with each broad category, they can anticipate and respond to these family dynamics in each new encounter. This collective wisdom of handling challenging encounters with families is invaluable to PGY-1 residents who are often unprepared and, as a result, are stressed by the interaction. It will not be possible to prepare for every difficult family encounter. However, learning how to systematically handle families and set appropriate boundaries in a positive way can help to minimize or prevent problems. For example, physicians skilled in family communication might be less likely to avoid challenging families, reducing the risk of missing important information that is related to patient care.

- **Listen actively and empathically.** "Active listening" means paying full attention when the family member is speaking, rather than thinking about what you are going to say next. It is important to listen actively to fully understand the person speaking. Often physicians let this skill lapse, especially when they are upset, do not understand why a family is making a certain choice, or are busy with multiple clinical responsibilities.

  Listening actively when families just need to vent and feel supported can ease a difficult situation and increase satisfaction with overall care. It can also help save time and lessen future problems. An empathic listener does the following:

  - Identifies the feeling that the patient or family member is experiencing
  - Identifies the cause of the feeling
  - Responds in a way that makes a connection between the two

- **Empower families by giving them some control.** Families often feel powerless and helpless when their loved one is ill. Having family-centered discussions and allowing patients and families to be involved with the treatment plan can provide the family with a sense of input and a degree of control. At times, families can be resistant to a treatment plan just because they feel powerless. For example, some families can be empowered by giving them small tasks to help with patient care, such as helping the nurses by monitoring blood pressure.

- **Encourage families to write their questions down.** Many medical terms and concepts come up during hospitalization, and overwhelmed patients and families will often think of questions only after meeting the physicians, and may try to contact the physician after rounds. Encouraging them to write down questions will help prevent confusion and disagreements and will assist physicians in managing their time more effectively. Educating families on disease processes and prognosis can help clarify treatment, ease anxiety, and prevent confusion.

- **Ask questions.** At times, patients and families will not communicate the reasons they are upset. They will be emotional and irritable during all interactions with the health care team, with perhaps only one underlying cause to their emotional reactions. It is helpful to inquire about the issue behind these reactions in order to help fix the problem. The inquiry method, in which gentle and probing questions are asked about what the other person is thinking and feeling, can be useful in this situation. The goal is to get the others to "lay their cards on the table" so you can deal with the problem and know where you stand.

  Sample questions: *"Can you tell me a little more about what is making you upset?"*

- **Stay aware of cultural diversity and be mindful of personal biases.** Patients and families come from different cultures and backgrounds with various life experiences and problems. It is important to consider these factors and have a professional attitude to lessen misunderstandings, disagreements, or conflicts. Try to put yourself in the family's shoes; treat the family as you would hope that a physician would treat your own family and loved ones.

- **Identify effective techniques to manage highly emotional family members.** It can be difficult when patients or their families behave rudely or angrily; however, it is important to stay professional in these situations. Responding in a defensive way is likely to worsen the situation. Residents can learn techniques to de-escalate intense emotional situations and manage hostility and conflict within a family setting. Using reframing techniques to understand that they are often upset and frightened with the circumstances, not at you, can help. The disarming technique, in which you find some truth in what the angry patient or family member is saying and acknowledge it, can be helpful.

If you feel you are getting overly upset and cannot effectively use these techniques, try to distance yourself by physically leaving for a short period to regroup and cool off. At times, another physician or nurse might already have a strong relationship with the family and can step in to defuse an escalation.

- **Formulate a plan for patient's discharge.** When the patient leaves the hospital, there should be a collaborative treatment plan and a process that includes all family members and the treatment team. In this meeting, patient and family responsibilities should be designated. The discharge plan should establish a clear role for family members, provide clear and realistic goals for treatment, and help clarify criteria that necessitates urgent intervention.

MedRAP Facilitator Manual

The curriculum for the Interacting with Patients' Families session can be found in this book on page 197. The manual includes detailed instructions for facilitators to conduct their own session on interacting with patients' families, as well as samples of handouts developed specifically for BCM based on feedback from the group leaders regarding ways to address specific challenges, facilitator input, and selected approaches from a wide range of leading researchers in different disciplines.

PRESENT REQUIREMENTS: ACGME COMPETENCIES ADDRESSED IN INTERACTION WITH PATIENTS' FAMILIES

Attention to family issues allows for the best integration of families into a patient's treatment plan. Communicating with families is instrumental to the assessment, alliance, and support of patients, and family-oriented patient care improves patient outcome and reduces family burden. Clinical family skills of communication that lead to improved understanding and rapport are part of ACGME's core competencies required of all residents.

Milestones Linked to Interpersonal and Communications Skills:

- Provide timely and comprehensive verbal and written communication to patients/advocates (ICS-A1)

- Effectively use verbal and nonverbal skills to create rapport with patients/ families (ICS-A2)

- Use communication skills to build a therapeutic relationship (ICS-A3)

- Engage patients/advocates in shared decision-making for uncomplicated diagnostic and therapeutic scenarios (ICS-A4)

- Utilize patient centered educational strategies (ICS-A5)

- Engage patient/advocates in shared decision-making for difficult, ambiguous, or controversial scenarios (ICS-A6)

- Appropriately counsel patients about the risks and benefits of tests and procedures, highlighting cost awareness and resource allocation (ICS-A7)

- Role model effective communication skills in challenging situations (ICS-A8)

- Effectively use an interpreter to engage patient in the clinical setting, including patient education (ICS-B1)

- Demonstrate sensitivity to differences in patients including but not limited to race, culture, gender, sexual orientation, socioeconomic status, literacy, and religious beliefs (ICS-B2)

- Actively seek to understand patient differences and views and reflects this in respectful communication and shared decision-making with the patient and the health care team (ICS-B3)

- Effectively communicate with other caregivers in order to maintain appropriate continuity during transitions of care (ICS-C1)

- Role model and teach effective communication with next caregivers during transitions of care (ICS-C2)

- Deliver appropriate, succinct, hypothesis-driven oral presentations (ICS-D1)

- Effectively communicate plan of care to all members of the health care team (ICS-D2)
- Engage in collaborative communication with all members of the health care team (ICS-D3)
- Request consultative services in an effective manner (ICS-E1)
- Clearly communicate the role of consultant to the patient, in support of the primary care relationship (ICS-E2)
- Communicate consultative recommendations to the referring team in an effective manner (ICS-E3)
- Provide legible, accurate, complete, and timely written communication that is congruent with medical standards (ICS-F1)
- Ensure succinct, relevant and patient-specific written communication (ICS-F2)

Milestones Linked to Professionalism:
- Document and report clinical information truthfully (P-A1)
- Accept personal errors and honestly acknowledge them (P-A3)
- Demonstrate empathy and compassion to all patients (P-B1)
- Demonstrate a commitment to relieve pain and suffering (P-B2)
- Provide support (physical, psychological, social and spiritual) for dying patients and their families (P-B3)
- Carry out timely interactions with colleagues, patients, and their designated caregivers (P-D2)
- Maintain appropriate professional relationships with patients, families and staff (P-F2)
- Recognize and address personal, psychological, and physical limitations that may affect professional performance (P-F4)
- Recognize the scope of his/her abilities and ask for supervision and assistance appropriately (P-F5)
- Recognize the need to assist colleagues in the provision of duties (P-F7)
- Recognize when it is necessary to advocate for individual patient needs (P-G1)
- Effectively advocate for individual patient needs (P-G2)
- Maintain patient confidentiality (P-J1)
- Recognize that disparities exist in health care among populations and that they may impact care of the patient (P-K1)

Milestones Linked to Systems-Based Practice:

- Negotiate patient-centered care among multiple care providers (SBP-A3)
- Reflect awareness of common socio-economic barriers that impact patient care (SBP-D1)

Milestones Liked to Practice-Based Learning and Improvement:

- Communicate risks and benefits to alternative to patients (PBLI-E3)
- Integrate clinical evidence, clinical context, and patient preferences into decision-making (PBLI-E4)
- Actively participate in teaching conferences (PBLI-H1)

Milestones Linked to Patient Care:

- Obtain relevant historical subtleties that inform and prioritize both differential diagnoses and diagnostic plans, including sensitive, complicated, and detailed information that may not often be volunteered by the patient (PC-A3)

Milestones Linked to Medical Knowledge:

- Demonstrate sufficient knowledge of socio-behavioral sciences including but not limited to health care economics, medical ethics and medical education (MK-A9)

The National Board of Medical Examiners (NBME) has also called for enhancements of the communication skills component of the Step 2 Clinical Skills (Step 2 CS), some of which were rolled out in June 2012.[18]

CHAPTER 13:

IMPROVING PATIENT-PHYSICIAN RELATIONSHIP

Effective patient-physician communication is essential to building good patient-doctor relationships. It has been reported to lead to better patient care, while lack of communication or miscommunications can compromise patient safety.[1] Current research suggests that ineffective patient-physician communication is one of the leading causes of medical errors, and breakdowns in communication are reported to be the underlying cause for about 80 percent of malpractice claims.[2] Studies have reported that as many as 15 percent of patient-physician encounters are rated as "difficult" by physicians.[2,3]

Difficulties with patients can be traced to several factors that may be related to patients (such as personality disorders and psychiatric disorders), physicians (such as overwork, poor communication skills, and biases), or the health care system (such as efficiency, effectiveness of care, and pressures to decrease costs). Patients who are described as difficult by health care professionals are likely to be depressed, have anxiety disorders or self-destructive tendencies, have reduced satisfaction as a result of unmet expectations, and have a tendency to over-utilize health care services. Physicians with poor psychosocial attitudes are more likely to describe encounters as difficult. Relationship difficulties develop when there is disappointment, unmet expectations, inflexibility, and unclear boundaries.[4]

Good interpersonal communication skills can vastly improve these difficult encounters. A variety of tactics and strategies can be applied to difficult encounters to reduce common physician-patient communication problems. Awareness of factors and preparing to address them ahead of time can greatly assist in managing and, at times, preventing miscommunication. It is important for physicians to be equipped with good empathic and interpersonal communication skills strategies.

Physicians cannot avoid difficult interactions with patients, but both physicians and patients can have better experiences when they have tools to deal with these challenging encounters as they arise. Both patients and physicians mention empathy as an important component of professionalism.[5]

Physicians benefit from well-developed empathic skills, which assist them in getting as much information as possible from the patient, and communication skills, which help in understanding, clarifying, and reflecting on the perception of a patient's thoughts and feelings.[5] Personality styles of "difficult" patients, described by health care professionals, include patients who are:[6-9]

- Dependent
- Denying
- Demanding
- Help-rejecting
- Emotionally needy
- Manipulative

It is important to remember that the label "difficult" can be subjective. Because individual experiences, perception and expertise vary, a patient labeled "difficult" by one physician may not be seen as problematic by another.

Physicians' barriers to good communication may include: stress, fatigue, and burnout; personal biases; language barriers; cross-cultural issues; and attitudes about care. Communication breakdowns that contribute to malpractice include encounters where:[3]

- Information is not clearly or effectively delivered
- Patient feels abandoned
- Patient senses devaluation
- Physician fails to understand patient's or family's perspectives

Improving physician communication and empathic skills can lead to:[10]

- Improved patient care and safety
- Increased patient satisfaction
- Better patient comprehension
- Patient's adherence to medical regiment
- Better diagnostics and outcomes
- A decrease in the likelihood of malpractice suits

It is important to address, develop, and reinforce these skills in the beginning of residency, when work habits are established. Residents can benefit greatly from the substantial research and information about patient-physician interaction. Residency is a very busy time with clinical responsibilities and workload. It is important to provide residents with information, best practices, strategies, and tips relevant to their experiences on the wards.

Empathic communication among medical students has been reported to decline when clinical rotations begin in the third year of training.[11] However, in a safe and positive training environment, empathy can be taught. When this is done, patient satisfaction and adherence to treatment improves and malpractice lawsuits are reduced. The development of cultural sensitivity and empathy fosters professionalism in residents, which is one of the ACGME competencies.

While medical schools prepare residents to solve medical problems and cure diseases, their graduates are often ill-equipped to deal with difficult encounters and patients' non-medical problems.[12,13] Such problems may include interaction with patients who visit their clinics frequently without apparent medical reason, are not motivated to improve, or engage in power struggles with health care providers.[14,15]

MEDRAP'S APPROACH TO COMMUNICATION WITH PATIENTS

MedRAP's approach to improving patient-physician interaction includes a focus on residents' biases. A carefully designed patient-physician interaction session, utilizing the process described previously and designed especially for the PGY-1 residents, can shape their work habits and communication skills in this formative year of their professional development.

Medical residents in academic centers typically interact the most with patients and are often first responders to patient management crises, giving them a unique opportunity to have a lasting impact. They have the power to permanently influence the way patients and their families experience, process, and remember a particularly difficult time in their lives: their hospital experience.

The residents' ability to effectively communicate with even the most difficult patients is essential for better patient care and satisfaction. Research suggests that residents tend to avoid patients they find difficult, and this avoidance could prevent early detection of a developing problem or the discovery of other vital information.[16] When residents accurately identify the characteristics of "difficult" patients, manage their interaction by utilizing effective communication strategies, and learn to set appropriate boundaries, they are able to more successfully interact with these "difficult" patients.

All doctors, however humane, will at times have negative feelings towards patients. Physicians have labeled patients as "difficult," "problem," "frustrating," "troublesome," or even "hateful." Emotional reactions cannot be wished away, nor is it good medicine to pretend they do not exist. The first step in managing difficult patients is to accept that negative feelings exist. Managing negative feelings towards patients may be difficult for residents, especially because of environmental circumstances, such as work overload, responsibility for multiple patients, stress, and burnout.

Maimonides, a physician who lived in the 12th century (1135-1204), wrote an oath and prayer for physicians: "May I never see in the patient anything but a fellow creature in pain."

Since compassion for patients is often a motivating factor in the decision to become a physician, residents tend to experience feelings of inadequacy, guilt, or self-loathing when they experience negative feelings. Acknowledging feelings of frustration or dislike of patients, and understanding that these feelings are "normal," provides relief. This acknowledgement is an important first step in managing negative emotions. If residents are trained to look deeper and identify the underlying factors behind the patient's negative characteristics (e.g. pain, fear, helplessness), or identify the causes of their own negative feelings (counter-transference), a place of greater understanding can be reached.

In order to improve the patients' and residents' experiences, impact patient care, assist GME programs to meet ACGME requirements, and help hospitals increase patient satisfaction, the MedRAP session format on patient-physician interaction sets the following goal and objectives:

PATIENT-PHYSICIAN INTERACTION SESSION GOALS AND OBJECTIVES

MAIN GOAL:

- To improve physician-patient interaction by meeting the following objectives:

OBJECTIVES:

- To present residents with foundational techniques, tips, and strategies for good patient-physician communication

- To help residents identify patients with whom they have difficulties communicating

- To assist residents in dealing with negative feelings towards patients through a self-reflection process

- To teach residents how to manage their own behaviors, feelings, and biases in these situations

- To introduce residents to categories of patients considered difficult by all health care professionals

- To provide strategies, best practices tips, and tools to manage challenging encounters with patients

STRATEGIES TO HELP IMPROVE PATIENT-PHYSICIAN COMMUNICATION[16-18]

Patients who are in emotional distress have various fears and anxieties that should be considered by physicians. These include:

- The impact of the disease on their independence
- The impact of the disease on their social life
- The nature and severity of their symptoms and associated pain
- The possibility of disability
- Disfigurement of their body and appearance
- Procedures they will have to undergo
- Death

Listen Actively

Active, reflective listening is a very simple but helpful patient communication tool. It helps patients talk constructively about their concerns; facilitates patients' ability to express deeper, less superficial thought processes; enables patients to discover some of their own answers and feelings; helps demonstrate the nonjudgmental understanding and concern of the clinician.

- Pay full attention to what the patient is saying so you can fully understand.
- Listen actively and truly understand the patient, which helps with addressing real concerns, improves adherence to treatment, and contributes to better care, thus reducing future problems.
- Generate questions based on what the patient says, rather than from a personal agenda.
- Summarize the patient's chief concerns and what you hear them saying.
- Reconcile conflicting views of the diagnosis or the seriousness of the condition.

Active Listening Process

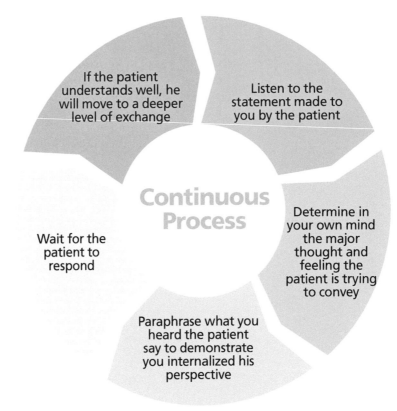

Continuous Process

- If the patient understands well, he will move to a deeper level of exchange
- Listen to the statement made to you by the patient
- Determine in your own mind the major thought and feeling the patient is trying to convey
- Paraphrase what you heard the patient say to demonstrate you internalized his perspective
- Wait for the patient to respond

Pay Attention to Your Non-Verbal Behavior

- Maintain eye contact.
- Nod to communicate understanding.
- Move closer to patient to share distress.
- Try to sit down to convey the message that you have ample time for the patient.

Elicit the Patient's Real Concerns

- Identify what the patient understands about the illness.
- Stay attuned to questioning style and non-verbal messages.
- It's often not *what* you say but *how* you say it that makes the difference.
- Make sure you communicate a partnership relationship.

Respond Empathically and Offer Support

- Demonstrate an understanding of the patient's distress and a realization of what the patient is going through.
- It is also helpful to state your personal support of the patient's concerns and struggles.

Beware of Personal Biases

Be aware of personal thoughts, biases, feelings, or stereotyping that may lead to unequal treatment. Some patients may interact in ways that seem:

- Overly cautious
- Resistant to recommendations
- Demanding
- Adversarial

These reactions may relate to patients' previous experiences with health care. Some clinicians may react defensively by getting angry, doing unnecessary studies, or overmedicating. Physicians need to understand these behaviors as responses to external factors. In addition, bias and stereotyping, although not necessarily conscious, may lead to unequal treatment.

Set Realistic Goals

Patients may come to the doctor with unrealistic expectations for a rapid diagnosis and a cure. However, the clinician may see this as a chronic illness requiring ongoing management. It is important to clarify goals and achieve consensus with the patient to avoid future disappointments about unmet goals.

Educate About Diagnosis and Prognosis

- Elicit the patient's understanding
- Address misunderstandings
- Provide information that is consistent with the patient's frame of reference or knowledge base
- Check patient's understanding of what was discussed

Provide Reassurance

In addition to patients' fear of serious consequences associated with their disease, they often feel vulnerable, out of control and helpless. The physician can reassure them by:

- Identifying the patient's concerns
- Validating and acknowledging them
- Responding to them

Negotiate Process of Care

Patient and physician must agree on diagnostic and treatment options. The doctor should provide choices that are consistent with the patient's preferences and interests in various treatments. Clarify the reason for the patient seeking care. Indicate what part the patient must play in caring for his or her health. Revise expectations if they are unrealistic.

Empower the Patient to Take Responsibility

Patients with chronic illness do better when they take responsibility for their care. The physician should encourage this and empower patients by preventing them from feeling helpless and dependent on the clinician, thus abrogating their responsibility.

Set Appropriate Boundaries

Some patients make unexpected visits, call frequently, may have a tendency toward lengthy visits, or have unrealistic expectations for care. It is important for the physician to establish and maintain boundaries and present expectations in a way that is not perceived as belittling or rejecting to the patient, yet is also consistent with the physician's personal needs to help prevent stress and burnout.

Work to Improve Patient Satisfaction

Patient satisfaction relates not only to the patient's perception of the doctor's technical competence, but also to the physician's humaneness, interest in psychosocial factors, and provision of relevant medical information.

PRESENT REQUIREMENTS: ACGME COMPETENCIES ADDRESSED IN IMPROVING PATIENT-PHYSICIAN RELATIONSHIP

Milestones Linked to Interpersonal and Communications Skills:

- Provide timely and comprehensive verbal and written communication to patients/advocates (ICS-A1)

- Effectively use verbal and nonverbal skills to create rapport with patients/families (ICS-A2)

- Use communication skills to build a therapeutic relationship (ICS-A3)

- Engage patients/advocates in shared decision-making for uncomplicated diagnostic and therapeutic scenarios (ICS-A4)

- Utilize patient centered educational strategies (ICS-A5)

- Engage patient/advocates in shared decision-making for difficult, ambiguous, or controversial scenarios (ICS-A6)

- Appropriately counsel patients about the risks and benefits of tests and procedures, highlighting cost awareness and resource allocation (ICS-A7)

- Role model effective communication skills in challenging situations (ICS-A8)

- Effectively use an interpreter to engage patient in the clinical setting, including patient education (ICS-B1)

- Demonstrate sensitivity to differences in patients including but not limited to race, culture, gender, sexual orientation, socioeconomic status, literacy, and religious beliefs (ICS-B2)

- Actively seek to understand patient differences and views and reflects this in respectful communication and shared decision-making with the patient and the health care team (ICS-B3)

- Effectively communicate with other caregivers in order to maintain appropriate continuity during transitions of care (ICS-C1)

- Role model and teach effective communication with next caregivers during transitions of care (ICS-C2)

- Deliver appropriate, succinct, hypothesis-driven oral presentations (ICS-D1)

- Effectively communicate plan of care to all members of the health care team (ICS-D2)

- Engage in collaborative communication with all members of the health care team (ICS-D3)

- Request consultative services in an effective manner (ICS-E1)

- Clearly communicate the role of consultant to the patient, in support of the primary care relationship (ICS-E2)

- Communicate consultative recommendations to the referring team in an effective manner (ICS-E3)
- Provide legible, accurate, complete, and timely written communication that is congruent with medical standards (ICS-F1)
- Ensure succinct, relevant and patient-specific written communication (ICS-F2)

Milestones Linked to Professionalism:
- Document and report clinical information truthfully (P-A1)
- Follow formal policies (P-A2)
- Accept personal errors and honestly acknowledge them (P-A3)
- Demonstrate empathy and compassion to all patients (P-B1)
- Demonstrate a commitment to relieve pain and suffering (P-B2)
- Provide support (physical, psychological, social and spiritual) for dying patients and their families (P-B3)
- Provide leadership for a team that respects patient dignity and autonomy (P-B4)
- Carry out timely interactions with colleagues, patients, and their designated caregivers (P-D2)
- Maintain appropriate professional relationships with patients, families and staff (P-F2)
- Recognize and address personal, psychological, and physical limitations that may affect professional performance (P-F4)
- Recognize the scope of his/her abilities and ask for supervision and assistance appropriately (P-F5)
- Recognize the need to assist colleagues in the provision of duties (P-F7)
- Recognize when it is necessary to advocate for individual patient needs (P-G1)
- Effectively advocate for individual patient needs (P-G2)
- Treat patients with dignity, civility and respect, regardless of race, culture, gender, ethnicity, age, or socioeconomic status (P-I1)
- Recognize and manage conflict when patient values differ from their own (P-I2)
- Maintain patient confidentiality (P-J1)
- Recognize that disparities exist in health care among populations and that they may impact care of the patient (P-K1)

Milestones Linked to Systems-Based Practice:

- Negotiate patient-centered care among multiple care providers (SBP-A3)
- Reflect awareness of common socio-economic barriers that impact patient care (SBP-D1)

Milestones Linked to Practice-Based Learning and Improvement:

- Communicate risks and benefits to alternative to patients (PBLI-E3)
- Integrate clinical evidence, clinical context, and patient preferences into decision-making (PBLI-E4)

Milestones Linked to Patient Care:

- Obtain relevant historical subtleties that inform and prioritize both differential diagnoses and diagnostic plans, including sensitive, complicated, and detailed information that may not often be volunteered by the patient (PC-A3)
- Customize care in the context of the patient's preferences and overall health (PC-F10)

Milestones Linked to Medical Knowledge:

- Demonstrate sufficient knowledge of socio-behavioral sciences including but not limited to health care economics, medical ethics and medical education (MK-A9)

The National Board of Medical Examiners (NBME) has also called for enhancements of the communication skills component of the Step 2 Clinical Skills (Step 2 CS), some of which were rolled out in June 2012.[19]

CHAPTER 14

BREAKING BAD NEWS

Breaking bad news is very stressful for most physicians, as well as their patients. Studies have shown that physicians who frequently give bad news suffer from higher levels of burnout. Physicians without sufficient training in breaking bad news experience great distress. Development of skills to deal with these difficult situations leads to more satisfaction among physicians as well.[1] Physicians who are competent and confident with giving bad news are perceived, by patients and families, as more trustworthy. Patients who trust their physicians are more likely to comply with treatment recommendations. Good communication skills are essential when communicating with patients with life-threatening illnesses.

Bad news is any information that negatively changes a person's expectations about the present and the future. News is defined as "bad" based on the patient's subjective perspective about the information.[2]

Doctors find delivering bad news to be particularly hard because they:[3]
- Fear the reaction of the patient and/or family
- Are uncertain about how to deal with the patient's emotional response
- Are reluctant to take hope away from the patient
- Feel like they've failed the patient
- Fear their own emotional reactions
- Worry they may be blamed for the bad news
- May be reminded of personal vulnerability to terminal illness or experiences of loss

While delivering bad news is difficult for all involved, fortunately substantial data is now available describing patient preferences in these interactions, the impact on physicians who participate in these conversations, and specific recommendations for the delivery of bad news. A specific skillset is helpful to communicate effectively in these challenging situations. Most physicians have little or no formal training for this task. Preparation for these conversations should be undertaken ahead of time in order to meet patients' needs. Familiarity with approaches to this process and incorporation of the key steps in these encounters will likely improve both patient and physician satisfaction, as well as patient care during these critical times.

Individual patient and family preferences for communication vary, so the best approach to delivering bad news should be tailored to each patient and diagnosis from the start of the interaction. For example: some patients like to have more detailed information, and some do not, and the physician needs to clarify this issue before beginning the discussion. Patients also differ in their reaction to bad news, and what it means to them can differ from patient to patient. For example, although all would agree that the diagnosis of cancer would qualify as "bad news," to some patients, discovering that they have hypertension could be devastating.

Effective strategies for the key issues of truth-telling, language, family involvement, and decision-making may help improve cross-cultural communication and understanding as well. Physicians should learn to address and consider cultural diversity issues. For example, some cultures believe that disclosure of bad news may cause patients to lose hope and give up.

It has been reported that non-English-speaking patients may receive less optimal end-of-life care than English-speaking patients.[4] Because language barriers may make a difficult situation even more complex, it is important to determine the patients' preferred language for prognosis discussions. It is recommended that a medical interpreter be present for discussions with patients and families, rather than depending on a family member to interpret.[5] This prevents the family member being the "bearer of bad news" and ensures an objective point of view in translation. The concept of autonomy is also important to consider when discussing bad news with patients and families from different cultures. It has been suggested that the Western value of autonomy, as practiced in the U.S., is not embraced by all cultures.

Tempering hope with realism is another great challenge for physicians. When bad news is delivered to patients, it often impacts their world and can change it forever. Hope can be a powerful force in helping with better adjustment, but it must be balanced with honesty and realistic goals. Several factors may allow patients to remain hopeful, despite a difficult prognosis, including:

- Fostering a good relationship between patient and physician
- Focusing on the potential for successful treatment
- Discussing the effects of the news on day-to-day living

Patients tend to prefer a realistic and individualized approach. In fact, the use of euphemisms and perceived unease of the provider actually decreases hope. Hope can also be facilitated by emphasizing what can be done, such as management of symptoms, and providing emotional and practical support in terms of daily life.[6]

Breaking bad news is one of the most challenging tasks in medical practice. Physicians are asked to undertake this unpleasant task at the time of a patient's greatest need. How physicians deliver bad news, their attitude, and communication skills play a critical role in how well the patient and the family will cope with it. There are good – and bad – ways to break bad news, and it is not always a function of experience.[2] Medical training should prepare young physicians to handle this duty carefully and systematically, especially since it has such an impact on patients, their families' adjustment, and physicians' well-being.

MEDRAP'S APPROACH TO BREAKING BAD NEWS

Many residents feel that they are inadequately prepared to deal with some of the most difficult tasks they face during the first year of residency, such as delivering bad news and talking about end-of-life care.[7] Studies confirm that residents have serious deficiencies in these areas.[7] While there is an increased trend in medical schools to teach these important communication skills with seminars and standardized patients, residents report this training is not always sufficient. Some of the reasons include:

- Communication skills are considered "soft skills" and are not assigned much importance.
- In medical school, clinical courses are considered more important.
- Medical students do not have the same level of responsibility toward the patient as the residents and do not usually break bad news.
- When these students start their residency and become directly responsible for patient care, they are confronted with various scenarios and realize they need help with delivering bad news.

Residents are exposed to the dreaded and uncomfortable fact of life: death at a relatively young age. They are hurled into the lives of terminally ill patients with very sad circumstances. To cope with it, defenses are raised that preserve the physician's capabilities for continued training. Utilizing these defenses helps young physicians insulate or distance themselves from the sad reality and mortality's implications in their own lives.

In order for residents to be effective in delivering bad news to their patients, the MedRAP curriculum deals with the subject in two ways: (1) technically, by providing them with helpful protocols; and (2) on a more personal level by self-reflecting on their personal experiences with bad news and its impact on them. If they cannot understand and analyze what they are going through when breaking bad news, it will be more difficult for them to be effective with their patients. They need to know what the bad news means to them. For example, a resident may encounter a medical situation similar to an event in the physician's own family, triggering an emotional reaction that can either help or interfere when communicating with patients and families. In general, delivering bad news is a difficult task for them, and they need to also learn to protect themselves while learning to respond empathically and companionably, in a way that communicates an understanding of the patient's feelings while maintaining appropriate professional boundaries. Without these boundaries, physicians can experience burnout or shut down emotionally. They need to learn to separate themselves from the patients and their families in a healthy way.[8,9]

Expressing empathy assists greatly in effective communication with patients. Empathy is often incorrectly conflated with sympathy.

- "Empathy is a complex affective and cognitive process of feeling, imagining, thinking and somatically sensing one's way into the experience of another person. The capacity for empathy lies at the heart of our ability to understand other people."[2]

- Expressing sympathy ("feeling with") can imply that the doctor is pitying or feeling sorry for patients, which can trigger a sense of inferiority and disempowerment.

- Expressing empathy is a more effective approach, as it places everyone on the same emotional level and does not convey a position of hierarchy, thereby helping to empower patients. Empathy demonstrates an understanding of the other person's thoughts and feelings, and provides reassurance that no judgements are being made. There are a number of ways in which empathy can be offered. For example:
  - Reflecting back to the patients feelings they expressed
  - Paraphrasing what the patients say to demonstrate understanding

In addition to the challenges described above, residents often have to deliver bad news to patients and families with whom they have no prior relationship, in settings that are not conducive to such intimate conversations. Their multiple clinical responsibilities may force them to have these important interactions with little preparation or when other medical emergencies are requiring their attention. MedRAP prepares PGY-1 residents to more effectively carry out these important duties by anticipating the needs for specific skills and providing the necessary tools, best practices, and relevant strategies.

BREAKING BAD NEWS SESSION GOALS AND OBJECTIVES

MAIN GOAL:

- To provide residents with strategies that will help them deliver bad news effectively by meeting the following objectives:

OBJECTIVES:

- To present general strategies and best practices

- To identify barriers to giving bad news to patients and family

- To help residents recognize their own personal difficulties and biases in providing bad news

- To provide tools to handle specific situations they are likely to encounter such as:

    - Breaking bad news over the phone

    - Breaking bad news of sudden death while being on night call

    - Asking for autopsy

    - Death pronouncement

    - Discussing difficult questions such as *"How long do I have?"*

IMPORTANT POINTS TO CONSIDER WHEN BREAKING BAD NEWS[10-13]

Maximizing the positive long-term outcomes for bad news recipients is challenging. It requires having a clear understanding of the goals of bad news transmission and strategies to facilitate their attainment. Burnout and poor mental health are more common among physicians who frequently give bad news. Physicians who feel unprepared for the task experience the greatest distress, and therefore it is important to be equipped with strategies to handle the disclosure.

Communicating the Information

- Patients should receive clear and honest information because it allows them to deal with the situation appropriately and plan for the future.
- The information provided should be consistent among patients and their family members to avoid mistrust.
- Knowing how much information to disclose is difficult, leading some to recommend that physicians repeatedly ask patients how much they want to know, thus allowing the patients to determine the level of information conveyed.
- In some cases, cultural, family, and personal preferences affect the amount of information patients wish to receive, and it is the physician's responsibility to consider these preferences.

Promoting Patients' Satisfaction

- Physicians can determine patients' preferences regarding delivery of bad news and use their responses to tailor the communication strategies.
- Information about treatment and prognosis is usually more important to patients than diagnostic information.
- Breaking bad news should be an ongoing process. Most patients cannot assimilate the information about prognosis and treatment options in one conversation. They need more than one interaction about the bad news to better understand what it means to them and to help them plan for the future.
- General expressions of support are very helpful to patients receiving bad news.

Improving Patients' Understanding

- It is important to give the facts in small chunks and check patients' understanding of the information provided. Some patients can experience "shut down" when they hear the word cancer and it is difficult for them to understand and remember the information they receive.
- In order to increase patients' satisfaction with the delivery of bad news, it is important to present the information in a way that patients can understand. For example, avoid using medical jargon.
- Different communication techniques can help patients better process bad news, such as active listening and reflection.
- To improve patients' and families' understanding, provide written materials and handouts they can refer to after the disclosure.

Reducing Patients' Distress

- Poor communication by physicians can worsen patients' distress.
- Patients' distress is most severe during and immediately following a bad news communication.

- Physicians' distress is most severe just prior to delivering the bad news.
- It is important to prepare in advance for the communication.
- Allow patients to express their emotions and help them put the situation in perspective.
- Acknowledge patients' distress, check the patients' needs and try to reassure them.

Promoting Hope

- Promoting hope as a goal for physicians can be problematic. It can have an impact on positive outcomes such as better adjustment, but it must be balanced with honesty and realistic goals.
- Factors that can increase the likelihood of promoting hope in a bad news delivery include: fostering a good relationship between patient and physician; focusing on the potential for successful treatment; discussing the effects of the news on daily life.
- Tempering hope with realism is especially important when there is a possibility that hope may be shattered at some point later, as is often the case during the course of a terminal illness.
- Hope can always be channeled toward improving some of the future outcomes or having a productive life despite the diagnosis.

PRESENT REQUIREMENTS: ACGME COMPETENCIES ADDRESSED IN BREAKING BAD NEWS

Milestones Linked to Interpersonal and Communications Skills:

- Provide timely and comprehensive verbal and written communication to patients/advocates (ICS-A1)

- Effectively use verbal and nonverbal skills to create rapport with patients/families (ICS-A2)

- Use communication skills to build a therapeutic relationship (ICS-A3)

- Engage patients/advocates in shared decision-making for uncomplicated diagnostic and therapeutic scenarios (ICS-A4)

- Utilize patient centered educational strategies (ICS-A5)

- Engage patient/advocates in shared decision-making for difficult, ambiguous, or controversial scenarios (ICS-A6)

- Appropriately counsel patients about the risks and benefits of tests and procedures, highlighting cost awareness and resource allocation (ICS-A7)

- Role model effective communication skills in challenging situations (ICS-A8)

- Effectively use an interpreter to engage patient in the clinical setting, including patient education (ICS-B1)

- Demonstrate sensitivity to differences in patients including but not limited to race, culture, gender, sexual orientation, socioeconomic status, literacy, and religious beliefs (ICS-B2)

- Actively seek to understand patient differences and views and reflects this in respectful communication and shared decision-making with the patient and the health care team (ICS-B3)

- Effectively communicate with other caregivers in order to maintain appropriate continuity during transitions of care (ICS-C1)

- Role model and teach effective communication with next caregivers during transitions of care (ICS-C2)

- Deliver appropriate, succinct, hypothesis-driven oral presentations (ICS-D1)

- Effectively communicate plan of care to all members of the health care team (ICS-D2)

- Engage in collaborative communication with all members of the health care team (ICS-D3)

- Request consultative services in an effective manner (ICS-E1)

- Clearly communicate the role of consultant to the patient, in support of the primary care relationship (ICS-E2)

- Communicate consultative recommendations to the referring team in an effective manner (ICS-E3)
- Provide legible, accurate, complete, and timely written communication that is congruent with medical standards (ICS-F1)
- Ensure succinct, relevant and patient-specific written communication (ICS-F2)

Milestones Linked to Professionalism:
- Demonstrate empathy and compassion to all patients (P-B1)
- Demonstrate a commitment to relieve pain and suffering (P-B2)
- Provide support (physical, psychological, social, and spiritual) for dying patients and their families (P-B3)
- Respond promptly and appropriately to clinical responsibilities including but not limited to calls and pages (P-D1)
- Carry out timely interactions with colleagues, patients, and their designated caregivers (P-D2)
- Recognize and manage obvious conflicts of interest, such as caring for family members and professional associates as patients (P-E1)
- Maintain appropriate professional relationships with patients, families, and staff (P-F2)
- Recognize and address personal, psychological, and physical limitations that may affect professional performance (P-F4)
- Recognize the scope of his/her abilities and ask for supervision and assistance appropriately (P-F5)
- Recognize the need to assist colleagues in the provision of duties (P-F7)
- Recognize when it is necessary to advocate for individual patient needs (P-G1)
- Effectively advocate for individual patient needs (P-G2)

Milestones Linked to Practice-Based Learning and Improvement:
- Communicate risks and benefits to alternative to patients (PBLI-E3)

CHAPTER 15:

CULTIVATING SYSTEMS-BASED PRACTICE SKILLS

The ACGME refers to providing affordable, quality care as "systems-based practice" (SBP), and includes it as a core competency for residents. The goal for this core competency is to help develop physicians who, in addition to providing excellent patient care, can participate in or lead constructive change in the quality and safety of the care delivery system throughout their careers.[1] The related ACGME milestones require that residents demonstrate the incorporation of patient safety and quality improvement skills into their daily activities.

SBP "focuses on the underpinnings of health care in a good medical practice: safety and quality in health care, physician advocacy, health insurance, health care economics, transitions of care, different health care systems, pay for performance, patient-centered medical home, and chronic care."[2] It reflects the need of the health care system to balance care and cost.

Systems-based practice (SBP) is defined as the ability to demonstrate an awareness of and responsiveness to the larger system of health care and the ability to effectively call on system resources to provide care that is of optimal value.

Health care financial pressures have continued to escalate in recent years, as costs increase and reimbursements decrease. Health care providers must continue to find ways to improve resource use and provide the quality of care that patients deserve, especially since they often pay the price of these demands.[3] Over the past few decades, dramatic changes in the practice of medicine have occurred without corresponding or matching adjustments in the health care system. As a result, both physicians and health care administrators have been frustrated and have had adversarial relationships at times, impacting health care outcomes[4]. Clinicians simply want to do their work unimpeded, providing high-quality, patient-oriented care. Health care administrators are responsible for overseeing the conditions that enable and promote quality care while factoring in limited resources as well.[4]

Physicians would like to perform their clinical duties independently, but their role as managers of care has diminished over the last few decades. They are faced with an administrative system that puts barriers and constraints in their way. They are often frustrated by a system that wants them to do social good works, but then puts obstacles in their way. They are often pressured by health care administrators who are responsible for providing care with limited resources, and at times do not understand the doctors' failure to operate within the parameters related to cost of care.

Physicians and health care administrators are both committed to the goal of providing quality care to patients at affordable costs. Their perceptions of each other and their resulting behaviors, however, may lead to misunderstandings and, at times, conflict. Health care administrators sometimes perceive physicians as naïve and unaware of the cost of care. Conversely, physicians sometimes perceive administrators as prioritizing their bottom line cost over patients. However, both physicians and administrators are committed to one common goal: good health care value for patients, which is the product of good outcomes and efficiency.

Both physicians and administrators want to provide value for the patient, and successful communication could help them work towards achieving this goal together by:

- Creating a positive work environment
- Improving care processes
- Ensuring that decisions are transparent and collaborative

Communication could be improved by increasing physicians' awareness of factors related to cost of care, involving them in finding ways to provide high-quality care while paying attention to efficiency. It is helpful for health care institutions to find ways to facilitate dialogues conducted to improve communication between physicians and administrators.

Physicians should be prepared to both deliver excellent patient care and to participate in or lead constructive change in the quality of health care delivery systems.[5] Better communication, collaboration and dialogue can also prepare residents for their future role in the health care industry. Structured dialogue can:

- Help physicians understand the complexity of hospital operations
- Give physicians and administrators the opportunity to discuss clinical priorities
- Improve communication between physicians and other health care team members

- Allow participants to identify inefficiencies, and recommend improvements in the hospital system

TO MEET THE ACGME REQUIREMENTS FOR SBP, RESIDENTS MUST BE ABLE TO:

- Work effectively in various health care delivery settings and systems relevant to their clinical specialty
- Coordinate care within the health care system
- Incorporate considerations of cost awareness and risk benefit analysis in patient or population-based care, as appropriate
- Advocate for quality patient care and optimal patient care systems
- Work in inter-professional teams to enhance patient safety and improve patient care quality
- Participate in identifying system errors and implementing potential solutions

MEDRAP'S APPROACH TO QUALITY IMPROVEMENT

Many educators report that it is difficult to meet the requirements for teaching the SBP competency. MedRAP's Quality Improvement (QI) method creates an avenue for structured dialogue between physicians, the health care team and hospital management. Specifically, the method allows residents to provide feedback on problems they observe in the hospital work environment and their residency program, and to suggest solutions to any problems that they encounter.

The QI method improves communication and collaboration between physicians and other members of the health care team by:

- Creating the opportunity to deal with issues early on
- Constructively addressing problems that arise in the system to improve the effectiveness and efficiency of clinical care
- Empowering the health care trainees and fostering a more positive organizational culture, contributing to better collaboration and effective and efficient care

The MedRAP QI method teaches residents techniques to identify systemic problems in the hospital work environment, then solve these problems through group brainstorming while factoring in the constraints of the health care system, such as limited financial resources. It is designed to elicit residents' confidential and anonymous feedback regarding their experiences in the hospital work environment. This feedback and potential solutions are presented to management so that the organization can take early action to improve the effectiveness and efficiency of patient care.

More than two decades of MedRAP data shows that implementing the suggested solutions from the QI presentations and resident feedback benefited the participating hospitals, leading to improved communication between health care teams, administration, and faculty.

The QI method is developed based on the principles of two organizational interventions: survey-feedback systems and quality control circles. These tools have been modified and tailored to the residency program, hospital training, and work environment, as explained in detail in the following chart.

SURVEY-FEEDBACK SYSTEM	QUALITY CONTROL CIRCLES[6]
Used to gather employee reactions and preferences so that management can take action to improve organizational effectiveness and employee satisfaction. Surveys are a systematic and thorough examination of the opinions, perceptions, and attitude of employees in the organization. They allow lower-level employees to anonymously pass on complaints and preferences. In a survey-feedback program, facilitators interpret the data from the questionnaires and lead small group discussions to examine the results. Survey-feedback programs are effective if they are: • Ongoing • Anonymous • Conducted by competent professionals • Compiled objectively and independently • Reflective of top management commitment to the process	A quality control circle is a management technique that encourages and teaches employees to solve organizational problems related to their own jobs. It is a participatory management approach. Employees meet in small groups to discuss organizational problems and issues related to quality productivity and to suggest solutions for improvements. The quality control circles are autonomous and are led by a supervisor or a facilitator. Participants receive training in formal problem-solving methods and then apply these methods to specific or general system/company problems. After completing the systematic analysis, findings are presented to management.

MEDRAP'S QI PROCESS

MedRAP's 4-month QI process begins with the systematic collection of data (through questionnaires). GLs and PGY-1 residents then conduct exercises to analyze the data, identify systematic problems, and suggest organizational improvements. Finally, the suggested solutions are organized, and the GLs present them to management in a formal setting.

SYSTEMATIC COLLECTION OF DATA

DATA ANALYSIS

ORGANIZATIONAL PROBLEM SOLVING

QI FOR THE RESIDENCY PROGRAM

PRESENTATIONS TO MANAGEMENT

The QI process introduces trainees to the entire quality control circle cycle, as well as more standard survey-feedback systems.

MedRAP recommends conducting the QI in December through March for several reasons:

- By December, the PGY-1s have already rotated through several rotations in affiliated hospital systems.
- By December, residents are no longer as overwhelmed as in the first months of their residency.
- January through March are known to be peak months for resident burnout. The MedRAP QI process empowers them to participate in bringing change to the hospital system and to their training program, which is associated with reduction in burnout levels.

Systematic Collection of Data
DECEMBER

December QI sessions are devoted to developing and updating questionnaires, administering them during the PGY-1 session, and conducting group discussions regarding the residents' overall program experience.

In the group leaders' (GLs') meeting:

- The GLs are divided into teams based on the affiliated hospitals. Together, they identify the most important systemic problems related to efficiency and effectiveness of patient care in the particular hospital system.
- The GLs develop and revise the previous year's questionnaires for their particular hospital, factoring in their specific observations. These questionnaires are used to measure PGY-1 residents' perceptions about every aspect of their training and patient care at the affiliated hospitals' training sites.
- A typical questionnaire asks the residents to grade their clinical and educational experience, within the affiliated hospital, on a 1 to 5 scale (1 = poor, 5 = superior). Some services evaluated include Ward Services, Consulting Services, Intensive Care Units, Facilities, Ancillary Services, Nursing Services, Social Workers' Assistance, Radiology, and Emergency Room. See next page for sample questionnaire components.

Sample Questionnaire Components

DEPARTMENT OF MEDICINE – MEDRAP
RESIDENT QUESTIONNAIRE

Please circle: PGY-1 resident   Senior resident

Grade your clinical and educational experience in the hospital
(1= poor, 5= superior)

A. Ward Services

Comments

1. Educational experience	1	2	3	4	5	_____
2. Teaching from GLs	1	2	3	4	5	_____
3. Attending rounds	1	2	3	4	5	_____
4. Quality of conferences	1	2	3	4	5	_____
5. Procedures	1	2	3	4	5	_____
6. Call schedule	1	2	3	4	5	_____
7. Back-up (when GL off)	1	2	3	4	5	_____
8. Efficiency of rounds	1	2	3	4	5	_____
9. Ability to attend conferences	1	2	3	4	5	_____
10. 80-hour requirement (Compliance)	1	2	3	4	5	_____

B. Interaction with Consult Services

1. Cardiology	1	2	3	4	5	_____
2. Gastroenterology	1	2	3	4	5	_____
3. Renal	1	2	3	4	5	_____
4. Infectious Disease	1	2	3	4	5	_____
5. Hematology/Oncology	1	2	3	4	5	_____
6. Surgery	1	2	3	4	5	_____
7. Others (please specify)	1	2	3	4	5	_____

C. Nursing Services (Wards)	Unit _____	Unit _____
1. Educational experience	1 2 3 4 5	1 2 3 4 5
2. Response to patients' needs	1 2 3 4 5	1 2 3 4 5
3. Attitude with residents	1 2 3 4 5	1 2 3 4 5
4. Knowledge of patients	1 2 3 4 5	1 2 3 4 5
5. Availability	1 2 3 4 5	1 2 3 4 5
6. Medication Errors	1 2 3 4 5	1 2 3 4 5
7. Attitude towards patients	1 2 3 4 5	1 2 3 4 5
8. Medical knowledge	1 2 3 4 5	1 2 3 4 5
9. Respect of residents' "protected time"	1 2 3 4 5	1 2 3 4 5

Comments

_____

_____

_____

_____

_____

In the PGY-1 session:
- Questionnaires are administered in December.
- This particular session also includes an open discussion about their overall feedback/experiences in the residency program regarding the first 6 months, including strengths and weaknesses of the residency program.
- Given the higher level of sensitivity of the December PGY-1 meeting, it is recommended that it be conducted offsite, in conjunction with a holiday lunch. Allowing residents to answer the questionnaires in a neutral environment can provide them with an additional sense of security, and they may be more likely to provide accurate feedback, even if the feedback is negative.
- Information from the questionnaires is tabulated to create tables of strengths and weaknesses for various services in the affiliated hospitals.

Analysis of Data
JANUARY

In the GLs' meeting:
- The GLs are divided into groups based on the hospitals they are assigned to; they review the questionnaire results for the hospital and identify the most important problems reported by PGY-1 residents. (See Figure 15-1)
- GLs are trained to facilitate organizational problem-solving by eliciting feedback from everyone, breaking problems into components, and solving problems under constraints. (See Table 15-1)

In the PGY-1 session:
- Residents are divided into groups – one group for each hospital evaluated – with a GL assigned to review and participate in the presentation of hospital improvements to the health care management team.
- The residents review the tables pertaining to each hospital. Using the tables as a guide, GLs identify additional difficulties encountered by the PGY-1 residents.

Figure 15-1: One example of data retrieved from a survey-feedback system and problem identification

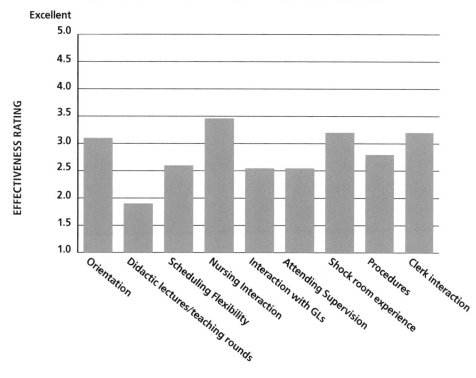

RESIDENTS' ASSESSMENT OF EMERGENCY ROOM ROTATION EXPERIENCE

HEALTH CARE TEAM SERVICES

Table 15-1

QUALITY CONTROL CIRCLES DEPARTMENT OF MEDICINE MEDRAP		
Identified Problem	**Problem Components**	**Suggested Solutions**

- The GL fills out a MedRAP-developed form identifying the problem, problem components, and suggested solutions based on the residents' feedback.
- Additional input on ongoing issues is collected to optimize potential solutions and to build consensus.
- The input from the different group sessions is compiled to be presented to all the PGY-1 groups for cumulative assessment in February.

Organizational Problem Solving
FEBRUARY

In the GLs' meeting:
- Teams of GLs assigned to each affiliated hospital evaluate the quality of all the suggestions generated at the January meeting, and select the important topics to be discussed with the PGY-1 residents and later presented to management of affiliated hospitals.
- GLs are chosen to present to hospital administration and health care team management.
- Each of these GLs is responsible for presenting the data along with the problems and suggested solutions.
- Facilitator assists the GLs in preparing for the presentation by:
  - Selecting the best solutions to present
  - Discussing relevant constraints and political issues
  - Choosing the most constructive way to phrase issues

- ◉ Assigning GLs to present a particular section
- ◉ Designing new tools/handouts for the presentation, such as "How to Optimize Patient Care with Admissions"
- ◉ Deciding which health care team members to invite

In the PGY-1 session:
- GLs review cumulative feedback of all groups and collect additional input.

QI for the Residency Program
MARCH

In the GLs' session:
- Questionnaire administered in December about strengths and weaknesses of the training program is analyzed
- The GLs prepare a presentation identifying strengths and weaknesses of the training program and suggested solutions for how to improve

In the PGY-1 session:
- The Residency program director attends the session and is presented with the data prepared by the GLs in the GL session. He responds to the ideas and suggested solutions.
- The program director updates the residents about changes for the next academic year.
- This process is intended to improve relationships between residents and residency program management, which contributes to improving residents' morale.

Presentations to Management
MARCH/APRIL

Presentation to hospital and health care team management:
- QI PowerPoint presentations are usually conducted annually in April. The presenting GLs team meets for several hours with the affiliated hospital administration and health care team management to present the findings, suggested solutions, and formulate realistic action plans for change in each affiliated hospital. In addition, the residents have an opportunity to hear the staff perspectives and learn if they can help them perform their duties better. They also brainstorm with different managers of the health care team, such as heads of radiology, the emergency room, phlebotomy, nursing, and social work.

- After the group has full understanding of each other's constraints, they all find collaborative solutions that can contribute to an efficient work environment.
- The group develops long-term plans to address issues that cannot be resolved immediately.
- After the meeting, the GLs report to the PGY-1 resident groups about the presentations in the different hospitals.
- MedRAP QI has also been conducted outside the residency program with fellows and junior attending physicians.

Sample of identified problems:

ASSESSMENT OF PATIENT CARE
ACROSS NURSING UNITS IN THE SAME HOSPITAL

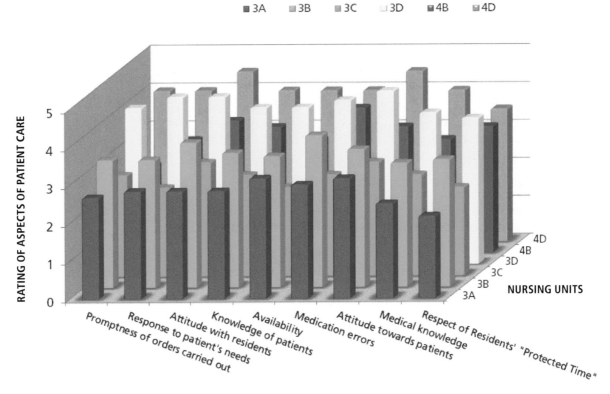

ASPECTS OF PATIENT CARE. 1= POOR 5= EXCELLENT

Samples of suggested solutions to Issues Identified in Assessment of Patient Care across Nursing Units in the Same Hospital

PROBLEM	SUGGESTED SOLUTIONS
1.) **Timely vital sign documentation and MD notification of abnormal vitals** • shifts missing • shifts recorded in nurse note and not in vitals section • MDs not always notified of abnormal vitals	1.) Implement systems shown to be effective in other units: • weekly meetings initiated by NU manager to discuss performance • NU managers round with teams to address concerns • Institute weekly meetings on all units • Encourage NU managers to ensure nursing duties are being appropriately done
2.) **I/Os, daily weights** • These are often requested and rarely done appropriately. This is crucial data that affects patient care.	2.) Implement consistent documentation: • Clearer accountability: nurse vs. tech • Recording vitals on white board by tech • Metrics in EMR to gauge compliance
3.) **Order delays** • Delays in ordering meds, labs, imaging in emergency situations on the floor because a physician must first place orders and sign them.	3.) Encourage acceptance of verbal orders through a set of clearly defined set of situations or criteria: • True emergency • Indisposed during procedure or with another patient
4.) **Communication with the PGY-1 resident on call ('the float')** • Many residents feel that RNs call without having necessary info ready (i.e. patient's team, current vitals).	4.) Implement a standard communication protocol which includes identification of the patient, the patient's team, the reason for admission, a current set of vitals, and current question/concern.
5.) **Clarification of capabilities of the medicine wards** • Certain meds/interventions are allowed on some units (eg: 3C v/s 3D) and not others. Clarify what can and cannot be done.	5.) Provide list of acceptable practices on each unit to avoid confusion and facilitate transfer to higher level of care when needed.
6.) **Differential performance and resident experience on different floors/units**	6.) Implement rating scale which allows differential unit ratings by residents. • Use data to identify problems with protocols or personnel • Identify "best practices" and enact in units lagging behind • Engage nursing leadership in evaluation process

The QI data can be utilized to compare performance across departments or units as described above.

The QI data can also measure trends over time, as demonstrated in the table below.

EFFECTIVENESS OF HOSPITAL WARD FUNCTIONS OVER A PERIOD OF TIME

WARD SERVICES

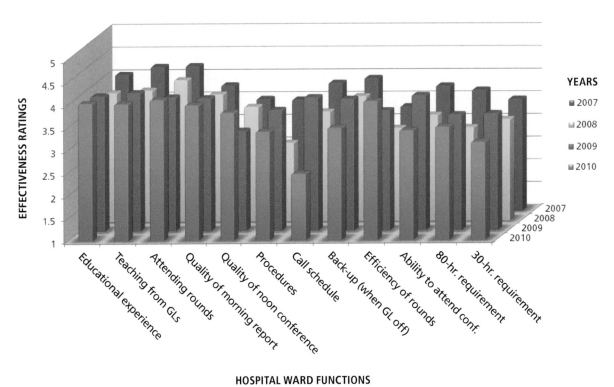

RESPONSIBILITIES THROUGHOUT THE QI PROCESS

FACILITATOR	GROUP LEADER
• Refine the questionnaires. • Lead the December session discussions. • Guide the GLs on conducting effective problem-solving sessions with the PGY-1 residents. • Review and select all the suggested solutions. • Prioritize presentation topics and refine the verbiage selected to ensure the message is communicated in a clear, constructive manner. • Instruct the GLs on presenting in a collaborative manner. • Invite the appropriate health care team members to the presentation. • Manage the overall communication and flow of the presentation, allowing for health care team member feedback and joint brainstorming. • Follow up with health care team management.	• Identify problems specific to a hospital system. • Help review and redesign participant questionnaire. • Work with groups of PGY-1 residents assigned to a specific hospital system, to identify problems with the system, quality, and efficiency of care. • Conduct brainstorming sessions with PGY-1 residents on organizational problem solving and identify solutions. • Review suggested solutions with facilitator and identify the most effective ones. • In conjunction with facilitator, prepare presentation to health care team management and hospital administration. • Conduct QI presentation based on facilitator guidance.

The QI process evaluates multiple resident experiences – from team hall to shock room in the affiliated hospitals – as well as the areas for improvement in the training program. This collaborative process improves morale and relationships between residents and management.

PRESENT REQUIREMENTS: ACGME COMPETENCIES MET IN SYSTEMS-BASED PRACTICE SESSION

Milestones Linked to Interpersonal and Communications Skills:

- Provide timely and comprehensive verbal and written communication to patients/advocates (ICS-A1)

- Effectively use verbal and nonverbal skills to create rapport with patients/families (ICS-A2)

- Use communication skills to build a therapeutic relationship (ICS-A3)

- Engage patients/advocates in shared decision-making for uncomplicated diagnostic and therapeutic scenarios (ICS-A4)

- Utilize patient centered educational strategies (ICS-A5)

- Engage patient/advocates in shared decision-making for difficult, ambiguous, or controversial scenarios (ICS-A6)

- Appropriately counsel patients about the risks and benefits of tests and procedures, highlighting cost awareness and resource allocation (ICS-A7)

- Role model effective communication skills in challenging situations (ICS-A8)

- Effectively use an interpreter to engage patient in the clinical setting, including patient education (ICS-B1)

- Demonstrate sensitivity to differences in patients including but not limited to race, culture, gender, sexual orientation, socioeconomic status, literacy, and religious beliefs (ICS-B2)

- Actively seek to understand patient differences and views and reflects this in respectful communication and shared decision-making with the patient and the health care team (ICS-B3)

- Effectively communicate with other caregivers in order to maintain appropriate continuity during transitions of care (ICS-C1)

- Role model and teach effective communication with next caregivers during transitions of care (ICS-C2)

- Deliver appropriate, succinct, hypothesis-driven oral presentations (ICS-D1)

- Effectively communicate plan of care to all members of the health care team (ICS-D2)

- Engage in collaborative communication with all members of the health care team (ICS-D3)

- Request consultative services in an effective manner (ICS-E1)

- Clearly communicate the role of consultant to the patient, in support of the primary care relationship (ICS-E2)

- Communicate consultative recommendations to the referring team in an effective manner (ICS-E3)
- Provide legible, accurate, complete, and timely written communication that is congruent with medical standards (ICS-F1)
- Ensure succinct, relevant and patient-specific written communication (ICS-F2)

Milestones Linked to Professionalism:
- Recognize and address personal, psychological, and physical limitations that may affect professional performance (P-F4)
- Recognize the scope of his/her abilities and ask for supervision and assistance appropriately (P-F5)
- Recognize the need to assist colleagues in the provision of duties (P-F7)
- Advocates for appropriate allocation of limited health care resources (P-K3)

Milestones Linked to Systems-Based Practice:
- Understand unique roles and services provided by local health care delivery systems (SBP-A1)
- Manage and coordinate care and care transitions across multiple delivery systems, including ambulatory, subacute, acute, rehabilitation and skilled nursing (SBP-A2)
- Negotiate patient-centered care among multiple care providers (SBP-A3)
- Appreciate roles of a variety of health care providers, including but not limited to consultants, therapists, nursed, home care workers, pharmacists, and social workers (SBP-B1)
- Work effectively as a member within the inter-professional team to ensure safe patient care (SBP-B2)
- Consider alternative solutions provided by other teammates (SBP-B3)
- Demonstrate how to manage the team by utilizing the skills and coordinating the activities of inter-professional team members (SBP-B4)
- Recognize health system forces that increase the risk for error including barriers to optimal care (SBP-C1)
- Identify, reflect on, and learn from critical incidents such as near misses and preventable medical errors (SBP-C2)
- Dialogue with care team members to identify risk for and prevention of medical error (SBP-C3)
- Understand the mechanisms for analysis and correction of systems errors (SBP-C4)
- Demonstrate ability to understand and engage in a system level quality improvement initiative (SBP-C5)

- Partner with other health care team professionals to identify, propose improvement opportunities within the system (SBP-C6)

- Reflect awareness of common socio-economic barriers that impact patient care (SBP-D1)

- Understand how cost-benefit analysis is applied to patient care (i.e. via principles of screening tests and the development of clinical guidelines (SBP-D2)

- Identify the role of various health care stakeholders including providers, suppliers, financiers, purchasers and consumers and their varied impact on the cost of and access to health care (SBP-D3)

- Understand coding and reimbursement principles (SBP-D4)

- Identify costs for common diagnostic or therapeutic tests (SBP-E1)

- Minimize unnecessary care including tests, procedures, therapies and ambulatory or hospital encounters (SBP-E2)

- Demonstrate the incorporation of cost-awareness principles into standard clinical judgments and decision-making (SBP-E3)

- Demonstrate the incorporation of cost-awareness principles into complex clinical scenarios (SBP-E4)

Milestones Linked to Practice-Based Learning and Improvement:

- Appreciate the responsibility to assess and improve care collectively for a panel of patients (PBLI-A1)

- Reflect on audit compared with local or national benchmarks and explore possible explanations for deficiencies, including doctor-related, system-related, and patient-related factors (PBLI-A3)

- Identify areas in resident's own practice and local system that can be changed to improve the processes and outcomes of care (PBLI-A4)

- Engage in a quality improvement intervention (PBLI-A5)

- Identify learning needs (clinical questions) as they emerge in patient care activities (PBLI-B1)

- Classify and precisely articulate clinical questions (PBLI-B2)

- Develop a system to track, pursue, and reflect on clinical questions (PBLI-B3)

- Access medical information resources to answer clinical questions and support decision making (PBLI-C1)

- Effectively and efficiently search NLM databases for original clinical research articles (PBLI-C2)

- Effectively and efficiently search evidence-based summary medical information resources (PBLI-C3)

- Independently appraise clinical guideline recommendations for bias and cost-benefit considerations (PBLI-D4)

- Respond welcomingly and productively to feedback from all members of the health care team including faculty, peer residents, students, nurses, allied health workers, patients and their advocates (PBLI-F1)

- Actively seek feedback from all members of the health care team (PBLI-F2)

- Reflect on feedback in developing plans for improvement (PBLI-F4)

- Maintain awareness of the situation in the moment, and respond to meet situational needs (PBLI-G1)

Milestones Linked to Medical Knowledge:

- Demonstrate sufficient knowledge of socio-behavioral sciences including but not limited to health care economics, medical ethics and medical education (MK-A9)

CHAPTER 16:

DEVELOPING EMOTIONALLY INTELLIGENT LEADERS

Physicians should have an important leadership role in health care organizations since they are at the center of clinical service delivery. Emerging evidence suggests that improving their leadership skills contributes to better outcomes for patients and for health care organizations.[1] In recent years, policy-makers and medical educators have shown interest in providing physicians with formal leadership training. They also recognize that the leadership skills of health care professionals can impact not only patient care, but also hospital efficiency and patient satisfaction, which is important to hospital reimbursement and overall cost of care.

The development of health care professionals' leadership skills has, traditionally, occurred randomly in medical training. Faculty and the curriculum focused primarily on instruction regarding critical patient situations, resuscitation, and technical skills, but they provided little formal training in essential leadership skills. With the changing health care industry, development of leadership in physicians is becoming increasingly important.[2]

Leadership training will be more effective if it first allows residents to: self-reflect; describe leaders they find effective or ineffective and why; and identify their own strengths, weaknesses, and areas for personal improvement when it comes to developing their leadership skills.

The majority of physicians possess the attributes most fundamental for leadership, such as strategic and tactical planning, persuasive communication, negotiation, effective decision-making, team building, conflict resolution, and interviewing. However, additional necessary skills require systematic training.

Traits such as intelligence, determination, and vision are necessary but still insufficient qualities to truly excel in leadership. Personal qualities are also essential. Although analytical and technical skills are required for a leader's success, studies demonstrate that emotional intelligence may be the most important attribute that distinguishes outstanding leadership performance.[3,4]

The concept of emotional intelligence ("EQ") is attributed to Professors Peter Salovey and John D. Mayer.[5] Psychologist and author Daniel Goleman brought the term to a wider audience with his book "Emotional Intelligence: Why It Can Matter More than IQ" (1995).[6] Today the concept of EQ is globally used. Truly effective leaders all have one thing in common--high levels of EQ. Without it, a person can have creative ideas, excellent training, and an analytical mind, but it does not necessarily mean he will make a great leader.[3]

EQ is defined as the ability to manage oneself in relationship with others, to recognize one's own feelings and those of others, and to manage emotions in relationships. EQ differs from cognitive intelligence (IQ). With IQ, people learn new facts, but their intelligence, or their ability to learn, is going to remain largely unchanged. In contrast, EQ can be taught and acquired. Studies conducted in industry found that all highly effective leaders have high levels of EQ.

The EQ framework can be very helpful in assisting self-reflection and insight into one's abilities as a leader, as well as in developing leadership skills. Goleman looked at three components and capabilities to analyze the performance of leaders:

1. Technical skills

2. Cognitive skills (IQ)

3. Competencies that demonstrated EQ

He found IQ and technical skills to be important, mostly as threshold capabilities and entry-level requirements for executive positions. He also found that the ratio of EQ as an element of success in high levels of management was twice as important as technical skills. He also concluded that EQ becomes increasingly important at the highest levels of management, and it seemed to be an essential ingredient of leadership. Fortunately, EQ is a soft skill that can be taught; people can actually increase their EQ by working on the specific skills and using self-reflection.[7]

Both organizational and clinical leadership skills are essential for addressing challenges faced by health care systems; however, many residency programs have not included sufficient clinical leadership training for residents. Although many clinicians develop leadership competencies through observation and on-the-job learning, this type of learning does not create great leaders. In order to develop leadership skills, residents also must be taught to self-reflect on their leadership styles, their strengths and weakness as leaders, team leadership abilities, or emotional intelligence as it relates to effective leadership.[3,8]

Residents become team leaders quickly – in their second year of training. In order to be effective, they need both organizational and leadership skills. Transitioning from the role of "heavily supervised" PGY-1 resident to a team leader is stressful for many residents, especially as their clinical and leadership responsibilities grow significantly. They are expected to undertake and assume many critical clinical roles, including leading multidisciplinary teams in a variety of medical settings. In many cases, they can move in a one-week period from being a subordinate in June (the end of the academic year) to being a team leader and a supervisor in July (the beginning of the new academic year).

Realizing the importance of developing leadership skills, some residents turn to leadership "capstone courses" that are provided as a learning modality by some specialty and medical organizations. It is not clear how effective they are, since there is not much published data about their impact.

Leadership skills can and should be developed in a systematic way for medical residents. It is important to identify best practices to develop the leadership skills of every physician in-training and help them identify:

- Leadership challenges they encounter
- Ways to address these challenges
- Their leadership styles

MEDRAP'S APPROACH TO DEVELOPING PERSONAL LEADERSHIP SKILLS

Based on feedback from the needs assessment, sessions on leadership development are timed to coincide with the PGY-1 residents' transition from internship to their second year of residency. Residents often report great levels of stress during this transition, as they become team leaders on the hospital wards and are expected to supervise PGY-1 residents, while their own clinical responsibilities significantly increase.

MedRAP's curriculum dedicates two sessions to this important topic. The first deals with development of awareness and self-reflection of their own strengths and weaknesses as leaders, exposure to different leadership styles, identifying their own style, and development of EQ skills essential to leadership. In this session, residents identify qualities that lead to effective and ineffective leadership, both in their supervising seniors and in themselves.

The second session, which is discussed in Chapter 17, deals with information specific to the individual hospital wards. It provides tips and tools to improve clinical leadership skills, including organizational skills, teaching tips, and ways to provide feedback.

MEDRAP EQ SESSION GOALS AND OBJECTIVES

MAIN GOAL:

◉ Help residents to improve their personal leadership styles by meeting the following objectives:

OBJECTIVES:

To identify:

◉ Valuable leadership traits

◉ Their own strengths and weaknesses as leaders

◉ Leadership styles and identify their own

◉ The EQ components that contribute to effective leadership

◉ Their strengths and weaknesses with respect to these competencies

◉ Leadership competencies that are important to effective performance in their residency program

◉ Their own strengths and areas for improvement related to these competencies

DEVELOPING EQ LEADERSHIP CAPABILITIES FOR RESIDENTS

The ability to manage oneself and one's relationships effectively depends mostly on the following EQ capabilities: self-awareness, self-management, social awareness, and social skill. Each EQ capability has specific corresponding traits and competencies as described by Daniel Goleman. Residents can hone their leadership skills and social competency by developing these capabilities. After learning about the EQ framework, participants identify their own strengths and weaknesses as they relate to these EQ capabilities. They formulate a plan to improve perceived areas of weakness, with the assistance of the group and the facilitator.

1. **Self-Awareness** - The ability to understand one's emotions and recognize their impact on work performance and relationships.

   Capabilities include:
   a) Understanding the connection between feelings and actions, and their impact on performance.
   b) Awareness and ability to realistically evaluate strengths and weaknesses, and to reflect upon and learn from experiences.

c) A strong and positive sense of self-worth and the ability to make sound decisions despite uncertainties and pressures.

2. **Self-Management** - The ability to manage emotional reactions to different situations and people, manage disruptive emotions and impulses effectively, display trustworthiness and integrity, and handle ambiguity and change.

Capabilities include:
a) The ability to manage feelings and emotions and stay focused under pressure
b) Demonstration of honesty and integrity
c) The ability to manage responsibilities
d) The ability to adjust to new situations, handle multiple demands, shift priorities, overcome obstacles, and generate new ideas
e) The drive to improve and meet internal standards of excellence
f) The pursuit of goals beyond what's expected or required and readiness to seize opportunities

3. **Social Awareness** - The ability to accurately read social and political currents, understand the forces that shape views and actions of people and organizations, and navigate politically.

Capabilities include:
a) The ability to understand what other people are thinking and feeling, understanding their perspective, and taking an active interest in their concerns
b) The ability to read the currents in the organization and build decision networks
c) The ability to recognize and meet patients' and families' needs

4. **Social skills** - Proficiency in managing relationships, communicating clearly, and handling conflict effectively.

Capabilities include:
a) The ability to take charge and inspire others, recognizing the need for change, removing barriers, and enlisting others in its pursuit
b) The ability to utilize persuasive tactics to build consensus and support
c) The ability to sense others' developmental needs, offering useful feedback, and offering assignments that challenge and foster a person's skills
d) The ability to deal with difficult issues in a straightforward manner, listen well, seek mutual understanding, foster open communication, and stay equally receptive to bad news and good news
e) The ability to initiate new ideas and move people in a new direction

f) The ability to resolve tense situations with diplomacy and tact; de-escalate disagreements and bring about effective resolutions

g) The ability to cultivate and maintain relationships that are mutually beneficial; build rapport and maintain personal friendships among work associates

h) The ability to build teams; pursue collective goals; model team qualities like respect, helpfulness, and cooperation; work with others toward shared goals

MISCONCEPTIONS ABOUT EQ:

- EQ does not mean just being nice; nor does it mean that expression of feelings should be unrestrained.
- The level of EQ is not fixed genetically.
- EQ is largely learned.
- EQ continues to develop as we progress through life.

MODELS OF LEADERSHIP STYLES[9,10]

It is important for effective leaders to be familiar with different leadership styles and to be able to switch styles as needed, when conditions dictate, in order to create the best organizational climate and optimize business performance.

- **Coercive:** This style provides a lot of instruction and can be perceived as micromanagement. It can be effective in certain situations, but it can obstruct flexibility and reduce employee motivation.
- **Authoritative:** An authoritative leader states the overall goal but gives people the freedom to choose their own means of achieving it.
- **Affiliative:** This style can be useful for developing teams and increasing morale, but at the same time, can allow poor performance to go uncorrected.
- **Democratic:** The democratic leader encourages flexibility and generation of new ideas, but can lead to delays in decision making and employee sense of lack of leadership.
- **Pacesetting:** A leader who sets high performance standards for himself and others positively impacts high-performing employees, but other employees can feel overwhelmed by such a leader's expectations and perceive him as being too demanding.
- **Coaching:** This style is effective when employees want to improve their performance and are aware of their weaknesses, but have difficulties changing their work habits.

PRESENT REQUIREMENTS: ACGME COMPETENCIES ADDRESSED IN DEVELOPING EMOTIONALLY INTELLIGENT LEADERS

Milestones Linked to Interpersonal and Communications Skills:

- Provide timely and comprehensive verbal and written communication to patients/advocates (ICS-A1)

- Effectively use verbal and nonverbal skills to create rapport with patients/families (ICS-A2)

- Use communication skills to build a therapeutic relationship (ICS-A3)

- Engage patients/advocates in shared decision-making for uncomplicated diagnostic and therapeutic scenarios (ICS-A4)

- Utilize patient centered educational strategies (ICS-A5)

- Engage patient/advocates in shared decision-making for difficult, ambiguous, or controversial scenarios (ICS-A6)

- Appropriately counsel patients about the risks and benefits of tests and procedures, highlighting cost awareness and resource allocation (ICS-A7)

- Role model effective communication skills in challenging situations (ICS-A8)

- Effectively use an interpreter to engage patient in the clinical setting, including patient education (ICS-B1)

- Demonstrate sensitivity to differences in patients including but not limited to race, culture, gender, sexual orientation, socioeconomic status, literacy, and religious beliefs (ICS-B2)

- Actively seek to understand patient differences and views and reflects this in respectful communication and shared decision-making with the patient and the health care team (ICS-B3)

- Effectively communicate with other caregivers in order to maintain appropriate continuity during transitions of care (ICS-C1)

- Role model and teach effective communication with next caregivers during transitions of care (ICS-C2)

- Deliver appropriate, succinct, hypothesis-driven oral presentations (ICS-D1)

- Effectively communicate plan of care to all members of the health care team (ICS-D2)

- Engage in collaborative communication with all members of the health care team (ICS-D3)

- Request consultative services in an effective manner (ICS-E1)

- Clearly communicate the role of consultant to the patient, in support of the primary care relationship (ICS-E2)

- Communicate consultative recommendations to the referring team in an effective manner (ICS-E3)
- Provide legible, accurate, complete, and timely written communication that is congruent with medical standards (ICS-F1)
- Ensure succinct, relevant and patient-specific written communication (ICS-F2)

Milestones Linked to Professionalism:
- Recognize and address personal, psychological, and physical limitations that may affect professional performance (P-F4)
- Recognize the scope of his/her abilities and ask for supervision and assistance appropriately (P-F5)
- Recognize the need to assist colleagues in the provision of duties (P-F7)

Milestones Linked to Practice-Based Learning and Improvement:
- Respond welcomingly and productively to feedback from all members of the health care team including faculty, peer residents, students, nurses, allied health workers, patients and their advocates (PBLI-F1)
- Reflect on feedback in developing plans for improvement (PBLI-F4)

CHAPTER 17:

STRATEGIES FOR EFFECTIVE TEAM MANAGEMENT

Preparing health care professionals for leadership roles has become progressively more important as the complexity of health care has increased in recent years. A great deal of health care is currently delivered by teams who must collaborate to ensure effective, efficient care and patient satisfaction. Failure in communication, collaboration, or team management often diminishes patients' experiences of care, health outcomes, and safety of care, while simultaneously increasing costs.[1] Physicians' leadership and management skills play an important role in their ability to deliver high-quality, effective, and efficient patient care, as they must decide what type of care to provide and manage its delivery.[2]

Most physicians are not formally trained in clinical leadership skills and these responsibilities are new and unexpected, in large part because medical schools and residency programs do not emphasize them. It is important to improve teamwork as part of the overall effort to improve health care. In recent years, physician educators and health care institution managers have recognized the importance of providing formal training in leadership skills to physicians. The ability to lead also impacts the experiences, learning, efficiency of subordinates and the health care team, and overall patient care. However, many young physicians report relying on observational, on-the-job learning and do not receive systematic leadership training.[3]

Clinical leadership is exhibited by practicing physicians when caring for patients in clinical settings. It impacts both quality and efficiency of care.

Leadership and management are both essential for organizations to achieve strategic objectives. They are closely related terms: "Management is defined as coping with complexity" whereas "Leadership is defined as coping with change."[4] Effective leaders demonstrate the ability to articulate a vision or goal, communicate this vision to others, build support for this vision, and empower others.

In order to function effectively and cohesively, team leaders should ensure that the team members respect and trust each other; understand the plan for patient treatment; understand the roles and tasks of team members and anticipate each other's needs; receive feedback on their performance; communicate well to accurately convey information; identify changes in the clinical situation; and finally, adjust strategies as needed.[5]

Effective leaders of health care teams are not top-down autocrats. Ideally, they enable teams by responding to needs of team members, develop them by fostering their capabilities, and coach them by providing developmental feedback. Team leaders need specific capabilities to help the team function effectively. They need to be able to create and sustain the conditions that enable the team to function effectively, to instruct the team on how to optimize its function, and to build the team's ability to accomplish its work and achieve its goals.[6-8]

Enabling the team includes:

- Forming and maintaining a clear understanding of team goals
- Establishing shared responsibility and accountability for achieving these goals
- Assuring that the team has adequate authority to perform its tasks
- Empowering the team members
- Keeping the team unified
- Coaching the team on how to optimize its performance

Developing the team includes:

- Administering effective orientations
- Establishing and communicating team's expected behaviors
- Ensuring a common conception of the team's approach to its work
- Fostering team collaboration so they can carry out operations effectively
- Facilitating a positive and safe working environment

Coaching the team includes:

- Collecting information on the performance of individual team members
- Collecting information on the performance of the team as a whole
- Evaluating team members' performance
- Providing constructive feedback

Characteristics of effective leaders include the ability to:

- Build a supportive culture that is open and encourages collaboration
- Exhibit commitment to individual and collective performance
- Set realistic expectations
- Treat failures as learning opportunities
- Avoid shaming subordinates for making mistakes
- Manage the team rather than individuals
- Lead team without micromanaging
- Provide timely, constructive feedback
- Maintain direct channels of communication
- Manage conflicts effectively

Effective teamwork is essential to providing safe patient care. It is important for the health care team leaders to understand that the health care team is more than the sum of the individual members, and that their role is to develop, coach and enable the team as a whole. Educational interventions can help in understanding the principles of teamwork and how to train teams to optimize their performance in the healthcare settings.

MEDRAP'S APPROACH TO DEVELOPING CLINICAL LEADERSHIP

The transition from the first to the second year of residency is quite challenging, as residents take on many new roles and clinical leadership responsibilities, including leading multidisciplinary clinical ward teams on general medical services and in the intensive care unit (ICU). Effective clinical leadership contributes to better medical outcomes, but few residency programs formally address this issue.[1] Many senior residents report feeling ill-prepared to lead teams effectively, which impacts the function of their subordinate residents, students, the entire health care team, and ultimately patient care. It is important to provide them with pertinent formal education and systematic approaches to help them build their effectiveness as team leaders.

Residents with strong management skill sets function more effectively in the hospital work environment and impart this useful information to their team members as well. Good management skills play a role in the quality and safety of patient services, particularly in large teaching hospitals and health systems. Crucial management functions include priority-setting to expedite patient services without the loss of quality of care; prioritizing while on call; and dealing with multiple, simultaneous emergencies. Importantly, these types of skills also reduce the potential for medical errors. Organizational skills for senior residents, tools, tips, best practices, and strategies are collected during the group leaders meeting, as well as examples of typical difficult situations they are likely to encounter.

Team leaders' performances vary, and senior residents develop best practices to orient, guide, supervise, provide feedback, and communicate with their team. These GL sessions provide the residents an opportunity to reflect on their experiences and discuss the effectiveness of the strategies, followed by selection of best practices that are then streamlined and transferred to PGY-1 residents in the form of handouts and different tools.

Experiential activities, including case studies that represent typical difficult situations, are utilized to provide the PGY-1 residents with opportunities to self-reflect in a supportive environment and prepare by developing their own specific strategies for responding. In order to develop the clinical team leadership skills of senior residents, a Survival Guide, developed by GLs utilizing their cumulative previous experiences, offers strategies and best practices. This handout includes: tips and tools the GLs found helpful on how to deal with the daily management of the team; conducting an effective orientation; setting appropriate expectations; conducting effective rounds; managing admissions from ER; interacting with consulting services; conducting effective discharge; utilizing time effectively to provide valuable teaching; awareness of common PGY-1 residents' medical mistakes; managing residents and students effectively.

Every GME training program has its special features and characteristics, and every affiliated hospital within the residency program has its unique challenges for team leaders. For best development of clinical leadership, the instruction should be tailored to the environment. Demonstrating to senior residents how clinical leadership skills would impact their performance as team leaders has been shown to be an important component of leadership training success.[9] Training programs that work best focus on clinical leadership in specific organizational environments, tailored to the needs of senior residents leading ward teams. Taking generic clinical leadership courses is less effective.[1]

In order to improve the clinical leadership of senior resident team leaders as they transition from internship year to second year of residency, and to assist GME programs in meeting ACGME requirements and helping hospitals to provide effective and efficient care to patients, the McdRAP session format on Strategies for Senior Residents sets the following goal and objectives:

STRATEGIES FOR SENIOR RESIDENTS SESSION GOALS AND OBJECTIVES

MAIN GOAL:

◉ To improve clinical leadership and team management skills of residents.

OBJECTIVES:

◉ To present residents with best practices, tips, and strategies for effective team management, including how to:

- ○ Orient and supervise new PGY-1 residents

- ○ Interact with attending physicians and other consultants

- ○ Plan effective rounds

- ○ Assist and utilize students

◉ To provide residents with techniques on giving constructive feedback

◉ To assist the residents in managing teaching responsibilities while running the busy ward team

◉ To present residents with typical challenges they are likely to encounter while leading teams and to provide useful strategies to handle them

STRATEGIES, TOOLS AND TIPS FOR EFFECTIVE CLINICAL LEADERSHIP

Giving Constructive Feedback

- One of the important skills this session develops is the ability to provide constructive feedback. Residents often have a difficult time providing feedback to their subordinates, which can create miscommunication and problems on the team. Providing constructive and corrective feedback is an important skill for supervisors. If provided in a timely manner, it can improve the performance of PGY-1 residents and can impact patient care.

- Subordinates should reflect on their action, act, and receive feedback on their performance in order to truly assimilate new knowledge. It is also important for supervisors to empower subordinates to provide feedback to them on how they can be more helpful to promote healthy communication and an optimal teaching environment.

- Miscommunications and unmet expectations have been correlated with increased levels of stress and burnout. Feedback can occur in an informal way in an ongoing manner during daily activities. However, there should also be time allocated to providing more general constructive feedback—for example, in the middle of the month—so that residents and students have an idea how the senior resident and the attending physician perceive their performance while they still have time to improve.

Some supervisors have difficulty providing corrective feedback because they have difficulty receiving it themselves. One of the major barriers to giving feedback is the reluctance to express negative feedback or constructive criticism. Some people are raised with the belief that they shouldn't hurt anyone's feelings, and that if they can't say anything nice, they should not say anything at all. As a result, supervisors may either avoid providing corrections to their staff, even when performance interferes with getting the work done properly, or do so in a subtle way that has no impact. At the other extreme are supervisors who state criticism with a fault-finding attitude, in vague terms with judgment and threats. To avoid either of these tendencies, it is helpful to provide senior resident team leaders with some useful guidance on how to give constructive feedback.

Feedback will likely be more effective when:
- Attention is called to a problem in a way that motivates the PGY-1 resident or student to correct it
- The PGY-1 residents or students know what needs to change
- There is input about what should be done about it

Constructive Feedback Process

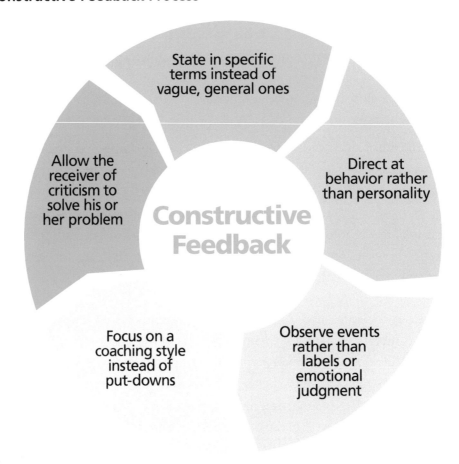

State in specific terms instead of vague, general ones

Allow the receiver of criticism to solve his or her problem

Constructive Feedback

Direct at behavior rather than personality

Focus on a coaching style instead of put-downs

Observe events rather than labels or emotional judgment

The Art of Teaching[10-12]

Another important competency the session develops is the ability to teach the junior residents and students in the busy clinical work environment. Senior residents find it especially difficult and frustrating to manage their teaching time and provide a good learning experience for their residents and students while also having so many new clinical responsibilities. It is important to provide them with tips, tools, and best practices on effective teaching.

In addition to case studies that deal with challenges they will encounter as teachers on the hospital ward, the PGY-1 residents are provided with tips and a collection of different strategies and best practices utilized by senior residents who are considered effective teachers. Some different teaching techniques include the following strategies:

- Deliver a brief lecture, when time permits, on essential topics that are not usually covered in morning report or noon conference.
- Write down important subjects to review at a later time with students/ PGY-1 residents.
  - ◉ Management of wound care (dressings and beds for different stages)

- ◉ Over the counter and herbal medications and their side effects
- ◉ Adult immunizations
- ◉ How to do a joint exam
- ◉ Review cardiac enzymes – which ones peak when, etc.
- ◉ Recent updates on how to treat cirrhosis, COPD, CHF, pneumonia, etc.
- ◉ How to interpret different lab results, e.g. LFTs, iron studies, TFTs, etc.
- Keep a small file folder of articles and old morning reports in the office.
- Prepare residents and students for their presentations on rounds; instruct them to be brief and to discuss only the pertinent points.
- Pace your teaching – there will be many daily opportunities for teaching but not all need to be acted on right away.
- Ask open-ended questions which allow assessment of the residents and students' knowledge base; tailor the teaching approach and prompt the learners to go into detail in their answers.
- Have residents and students make short presentations on topics of interest.
- Summarize what has been learned at the end of each day.
- Encourage everyone to ask questions.
- Don't be afraid to learn from your residents or to admit when you do not know something. People respect honesty.
- Keep up morale by:
  - ◉ Functioning as a team
  - ◉ Helping each other out
  - ◉ Helping the post-float person get out early
  - ◉ Try rounding on their new patients the afternoon of day call
  - ◉ Consider rounding with one PGY-1 resident so the other can get things done, especially if rounds are long
  - ◉ Minimizing negativity in front of the residents and students
  - ◉ Keeping snacks in your office; ordering out when on call

PRESENT REQUIREMENTS: ACGME COMPETENCIES MET IN STRATEGIES FOR EFFECTIVE TEAM MANAGEMENT

Milestones Linked to Interpersonal and Communications Skills:

- Provide timely and comprehensive verbal and written communication to patients/advocates (ICS-A1)
- Effectively use verbal and nonverbal skills to create rapport with patients/families (ICS-A2)
- Use communication skills to build a therapeutic relationship (ICS-A3)
- Engage patients/advocates in shared decision-making for uncomplicated diagnostic and therapeutic scenarios (ICS-A4)
- Utilize patient centered educational strategies (ICS-A5)
- Engage patient/advocates in shared decision-making for difficult, ambiguous, or controversial scenarios (ICS-A6)
- Appropriately counsel patients about the risks and benefits of tests and procedures, highlighting cost awareness and resource allocation (ICS-A7)
- Role model effective communication skills in challenging situations (ICS-A8)
- Effectively use an interpreter to engage patient in the clinical setting, including patient education (ICS-B1)
- Demonstrate sensitivity to differences in patients including but not limited to race, culture, gender, sexual orientation, socioeconomic status, literacy, and religious beliefs (ICS-B2)
- Actively seek to understand patient differences and views and reflects this in respectful communication and shared decision-making with the patient and the health care team (ICS-B3)
- Effectively communicate with other caregivers in order to maintain appropriate continuity during transitions of care (ICS-C1)
- Role model and teach effective communication with next caregivers during transitions of care (ICS-C2)
- Deliver appropriate, succinct, hypothesis-driven oral presentations (ICS-D1)
- Effectively communicate plan of care to all members of the health care team (ICS-D2)
- Engage in collaborative communication with all members of the health care team (ICS-D3)
- Request consultative services in an effective manner (ICS-E1)
- Clearly communicate the role of consultant to the patient, in support of the primary care relationship (ICS-E2)

- Communicate consultative recommendations to the referring team in an effective manner (ICS-E3)
- Provide legible, accurate, complete, and timely written communication that is congruent with medical standards (ICS-F1)
- Ensure succinct, relevant and patient-specific written communication (ICS-F2)

Milestones Linked to Professionalism:

- Follow formal policies (P-A2)
- Accept personal errors and honestly acknowledge them (P-A3)
- Provide leadership for a team that respects patient dignity and autonomy (P-B4)
- Respond promptly and appropriately to clinical responsibilities including but not limited to calls and pages (P-D1)
- Carry out timely interactions with colleagues, patients, and their designated caregivers (P-D2)
- Recognize and manage obvious conflicts of interest, such as caring for family members and professional associates as patients (P-E1)
- Maintain appropriate professional relationships with patients, families, and staff (P-F2)
- Ensure prompt completion of clinical, administrative, and curricular tasks (P-F3)
- Recognize and address personal, psychological, and physical limitations that may affect professional performance (P-F4)
- Recognize the scope of his/her abilities and ask for supervision and assistance appropriately (P-F5)
- Serve as a professional role model for more junior colleagues (e.g. medical students, interns) (P-F6)
- Recognize the need to assist colleagues in the provision of duties (P-F7)
- Recognize when it is necessary to advocate for individual patient needs (P-G1)
- Educate and hold others accountable for patient confidentiality (P-J2)

Milestones Linked to Systems-Based Practice:

- Understand unique roles and services provided by local health care delivery systems (SBP-A1)
- Manage and coordinate care and care transitions across multiple delivery systems, including ambulatory, subacute, acute, rehabilitation, and skilled nursing (SBP-A2)
- Negotiate patient-centered care among multiple care providers (SBP-A3)
- Appreciate roles of a variety of health care providers, including but not limited

to consultants, therapists, nurses, home care workers, pharmacists, and social workers (SBP-B1)

- Work effectively as a member within the inter professional team to ensure safe patient care (SBP-B2)
- Consider alternative solutions provided by other teammates (SBP-B3)
- Demonstrate how to manage the team by utilizing the skills and coordinating the activities of inter professional team members (SBP-B4)
- Identify, reflect on, and learn from critical incidents such as near misses and preventable medical errors (SBP-C2)
- Dialogue with care team members to identify risk for and prevention of medical error (SBP-C3)

Milestones Linked to Practice-Based Learning and Improvement:

- Identify learning needs (clinical questions) as they emerge in patient care activities (PBLI-B1)
- Classify and precisely articulate clinical questions (PBLI-B2)
- Develop a system to track, pursue, and reflect on clinical questions (PBLI-B3)
- Access medical information resources to answer clinical questions and support decision making (PBLI-C1)
- Effectively and efficiently search NLM databases for original clinical research articles (PBLI-C2)
- Effectively and efficiently search evidence-based summary medical information resources (PBLI-C3)
- Appraise the quality of medical information resources and select among them based on the characteristics of the clinical question (PBLI-C4)
- Communicate risks, benefits, and alternative treatment to patients (PBLI-E3)
- Respond welcomingly and productively to feedback from all members of the health care team, including faculty, peer residents, students, nurses, allied health workers, patients, and their advocates (PBLI-F1)
- Actively seek feedback from all members of the health care team (PBLI-F2)
- Calibrate self-assessment with feedback and other external data (PBLI-F3)
- Reflect on feedback in developing plans for improvement (PBLI-F4)
- Maintain awareness of the situation in the moment, and respond to meet situational needs (PBLI-G1)
- Reflect (in action) when surprised, applies new insights to future clinical scenarios, and reflects (on action) back on the process (PBLI-G2)
- Actively participate in teaching conferences (PBLI-H1)

- Integrate teaching, feedback, and evaluation with supervision of interns' and students' patient care (PBLI-H2)
- Take a leadership role in the education of all members of the health care team (PBLI-H3)

Milestones Linked to Patient Care:

- Seek and obtain appropriate, verified, and prioritized data from secondary sources (e.g. family, records, pharmacy) (PC-A2)
- Role model gathering subtle and reliable information from the patient for junior members of the health care team (PC-A4)
- Recognize situations with a need for a need for urgent or emergent medical care, including life-threatening conditions (PC-F1)
- Recognize when to seek additional guidance (PC-F2)
- Initiate management and stabilize patients with emergent medical conditions (PC-F6)

Milestones Linked to Medical Knowledge:

- Demonstrate sufficient knowledge of socio-behavioral sciences including but not limited to health care economics, medical ethics and medical education (MK-A9)

SECTION 5

PROGRAM EVALUATION AND LOOKING TO THE FUTURE

The following section presents data collected regarding MedRAP's success in achieving its goals. This section also discusses lessons learned, benefits of the MedRAP program, and its applicability to other health care professionals.

CHAPTER 18:

PROGRAM EVALUATION AND EVOLUTION

In addition to the monthly evaluations conducted at every GL meeting, the facilitators have conducted an annual needs assessment and analysis since the inception of the program (see Table 18-1). The results help to formulate the subsequent year's session schedule, decide on the key topics to be covered, and incorporate new challenges the residents are likely to face.

The MedRAP evaluation measures the degree to which 10 identified goals have been achieved, utilizing a 5-level Likert scale with anchors ranging from "low degree" (1) to "high degree" (5). A score of 2 or lower is defined as low success (LS) and a score of 4 or higher as high success (HS). The questionnaire also includes free text questions which ask respondents about the program's strengths and weaknesses.

Table 18-1: MedRAP Residents' Annual Evaluation

E) Please rate on a scale of 1-5: To what degree did the MedRAP Resident Assistance Program achieve the following goals?

```
|-------------|-----------|-----------|-------------|
1             2           3           4           5
Low                                               High
Degree                                          Degree
```

GOALS	RATINGS
1. Help you function more effectively in the system	1 2 3 4 5
2. Accelerate adaptation process to the internship year	1 2 3 4 5
3. Provide you with peer support	1 2 3 4 5
4. Identify elements of internship stress	1 2 3 4 5
5. Help you acquire effective coping strategies (In dealing with patients, their families, DNR situation)	1 2 3 4 5
6. Discuss issues of professional competency and identity	1 2 3 4 5
7. Improve communication with other residents	1 2 3 4 5
8. Improve communication with upper level residents	1 2 3 4 5
9. Improve the way you relate to your patients and their families	1 2 3 4 5
10. Contribute to your overall future role as a team leader	1 2 3 4 5

Figure 18-1 represents annual evaluation data collected at three points of time over two decades.

Figure 18-1: MedRAP's Success in Achieving Goals in 10-Year Increments

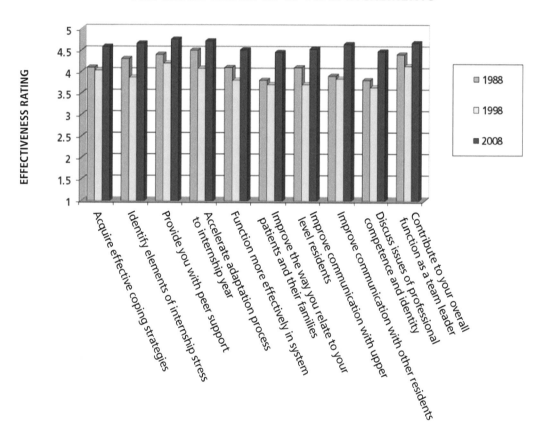

ASSESSMENT OF MEDRAP IN ACHIEVING PROGRAM GOALS IN 10-YEAR INCREMENTS

MEDRAP PROGRAM GOALS

Table 18-2 shows annual evaluation data over a 10-year period for PGY-1 resident respondents (N=458). The annual evaluation was designed to assess factors in the areas of professionalism and burnout. Residents reported that MedRAP achieved High Score (HS) across all goals, with mean HS rate for factors related to burnout reduction (91.4%; 95% CI, 90.2%-92.5%) and improved professionalism (87.4%; 95% CI, 86.0%-88.7%). Goals with HS rates above 90% were helping PGY-1 residents to function effectively, accelerate their adaptation, identify stressful elements, prepare for future role as team leaders, and receive peer support.

Table 18-2: Analysis of Responses to MedRAP Annual Evaluation

	# Responses	Responses				
		1	2	3	4	5
Burnout	457	0 (0%)	4 (1%)	35 (8%)	179 (39%)	239 (52%)
Function effectively in work environment	458	0 (0%)	6 (1%)	38 (8%)	232 (51%)	182 (40%)
Accelerate adaptation to internship	457	1 (0%)	3 (1%)	39 (9%)	190 (42%)	224 (49%)
Identify elements of internship stress	456	0 (0%)	3 (1%)	21 (5%)	152 (33%)	280 (61%)
Acquire effective coping strategies	458	0 (0%)	5 (1%)	51 (11%)	206 (45%)	196 (43%)
Provide peer support	458	1 (0%)	3 (1%)	24 (5%)	115 (25%)	315 (69%)
Professionalism	456	0 (0%)	5 (1%)	52 (11%)	193 (42%)	206 (45%)
Contribute to future function as team leader	455	0 (0%)	1 (0%)	27 (6%)	176 (39%)	251 (55%)
Discuss competence and identity issues	457	0 (0%)	7 (2%)	45 (10%)	214 (47%)	191 (42%)
Improve communication with residents	456	0 (0%)	6 (1%)	69 (15%)	182 (40%)	199 (44%)
Improve communication with UL residents	456	0 (0%)	4 (1%)	54 (12%)	176 (39%)	222 (49%)
Improve communication with patients / families	455	1 (0%)	7 (2%)	63 (14%)	216 (47%)	168 (37%)

Figure 18-2 and Figure 18-3 provide additional evaluation data, grouped by professional development and stress/burnout reduction, respectively. Data was pulled for three years, each a decade apart, in order to show an unbiased snapshot of the program at three points in time.

Figure 18-2: MedRAP's Impact on Factors in Contributing to Professional Development

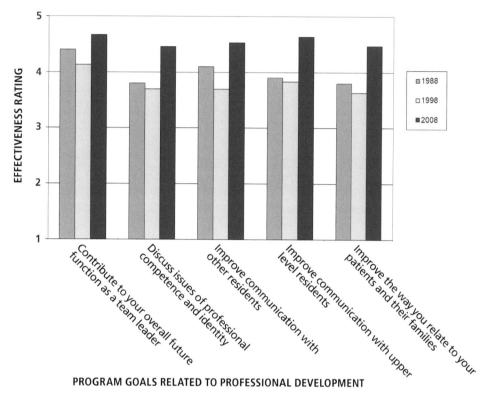

ASSESSMENT OF MEDRAP PROGRAM GOALS RELATED TO PROFESSIONAL DEVEOPMENT

PROGRAM GOALS RELATED TO PROFESSIONAL DEVELOPMENT

Figure 18-3: MedRAP's Impact on Factors Contributing to Stress and Burnout Reduction

ASSESSMENT OF MEDRAP PROGRAM GOALS RELATED TO BURNOUT

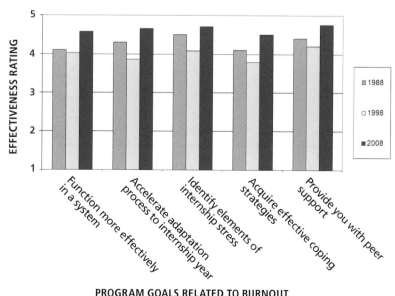

PROGRAM GOALS RELATED TO BURNOUT

OTHER FORMS OF EVALUATION

Below is data collected from residents in July 2010, at the beginning of residency, and in February 2011, midway through the year. Research indicates that residents' levels of stress and burnout traditionally peak in January and February during the academic year. Responses of MedRAP participants in the chart below suggest that the residents had more positive feelings about their program in February than they did in the beginning of the year. These responses suggest high morale, correlated with reduced levels of burnout. Participants responded to the following questions:

How confident are you that the residents in your program can:

1. Maintain a high level of morale?   1 2 3 4 5 6

2. Provide each other with peer support?   1 2 3 4 5 6

3. Have a supportive relationship with your upper level residents?   1 2 3 4 5 6

4. Communicate concerns to each other?   1 2 3 4 5 6

5. Resolve interpersonal conflicts?   1 2 3 4 5 6

6. Provide ongoing feedback about their educational experience without fear of retaliation?   1 2 3 4 5 6

7. Bring about organizational change to their program?   1 2 3 4 5 6

8. Improve the quality of your educational experience?   1 2 3 4 5 6

9. Utilize effective techniques for organizational problem solving?   1 2 3 4 5 6

10 Effectively discuss organizational change in a collaborative fashion with program directors?   1 2 3 4 5 6

11. Improve the efficiency of the hospital work environment?   1 2 3 4 5 6

ASSESSMENT OF TRAINING ENVIRONMENT,
ACADEMIC YEAR 2010-2011

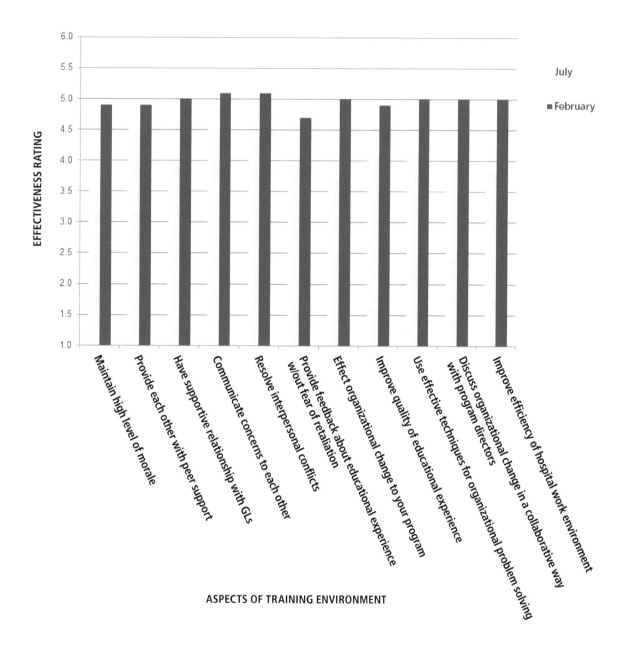

PARTICIPANTS' TESTIMONIALS

The annual evaluation questionnaire also contained specific open-ended questions to assess ways to improve the program. Below is a sample of responses.

"This is an excellent program: I am incredibly appreciative of everyone's hard work to help us. I hope the program never changes."

"I enjoyed being a group leader; I feel that the MedRAP program is one of the strongest aspects of our program."

"So glad this was a part of internship; it was a very valuable experience."

"I found the MedRAP meetings to be incredibly useful and filled me with great perspective. I think MedRAP is one of the finest things Baylor provides for us and felt lucky to be at an institution that really works hard to ensure all its members are both physically and mentally doing well."

"The program contributed to culture change in the department and system level change in the hospitals."

"Overall great experience. Maybe meet with only interns at some point or meet with interns individually once or twice a year."

"Hearing about other residents struggling to work efficiently. Getting advice from upper levels. Being able to have a mechanism for translating feedback into changes."

"Overall a great program and a tremendous asset for the residents/interns."

"Thanks! This program is an excellent way to help the transition through intern year and residency. MedRAP is truly one of the best aspects of our residency program."

MANAGEMENT TESTIMONIALS

Through the years MedRAP has received feedback from training program and departmental management. Below is a sample of responses.

"For the past 20 years, one of the strongest aspects of the internal medicine residency program has been the Resident Assistance Program. Because of this program, we are able to perform effective quality assurance functions, and provide personal counseling and a forum for constructive venting. In addition,

the program is a very valuable means of fulfilling a number of the ACGME competencies. One of the reasons that this program works so effectively is the dedication of the upper level residents who work closely with Iris Mushin to provide critical structure and experience for our interns."

- Director, Residency Programs in Internal Medicine,
Baylor College of Medicine

"The resident assistance program (MedRAP) of the Department of Medicine has been very effective in maintaining and improving the morale of our residents, while at the same time providing an opportunity to develop constructive solutions to efficiency and quality of care issues that affect the working environment at our affiliate hospitals."

- Chairman, Department of Medicine,
Baylor College of Medicine

"The Resident Assistance Program has been an invaluable part of our internal medicine training program for the past 22 years. As a program director, the benefits I see in this program are many and long lasting. As an independent and integrated program, it meets not only the residents' needs, but also supports the management of institutional and academic goals.

"Through the years, I have also received feedback from different health care team members who have felt that the program contributed to improved collaboration and thus improved patient care. I have been discussing the program in my presentations to new applicants and feel it is a great asset to our recruitment process."

- Associate Professor of Medicine and Medical Ethics,
Baylor College of Medicine

SUMMARY OF MAJOR THEMES REFLECTED IN MEDRAP ANNUAL EVALUATION

There were common themes and significant benefits reported by MedRAP participants. According to evaluations, the program:

- Successfully anticipated many difficult situations they encountered.
- Provided them with effective insight and strategies to deal with such situations.

- Allowed for a variety of problems to be considered because of the highly structured nature of the sessions.
- Maintained structured sessions that effectively prevented them from being gripe sessions, thus maintaining their problem-solving orientation.
- Reportedly accelerated learning, utilizing methods of sharing experiences, self-reflection, learning from peers, and mentorship from senior residents, all conducted in a confidential setting.

The collected data of the program suggested that it is possible to anticipate some of the difficult situations residents commonly encounter. This seems to be the result of careful analysis of topics and breaking down of problems into components relevant to the institution.

The senior residents serving as group leaders also benefited from their participation. They reported:

- Becoming more sympathetic to PGY-1 residents' experiences, which led to improved relations between junior and senior residents in the department
- Improving their leadership skills
- Feeling empowered to be part of the QI

Another measurement of the success of the program was the participation rate. An average of 80%-90% of PGY-1 residents actively participated in the MedRAP program over the years, attending about 70% of the sessions—despite its voluntary nature. They came to the sessions from four affiliated hospitals; coming to the meeting meant, on average, an additional 1-2 hours of work for the day.

MEDRAP BENEFITS REPORTED IN THE PILOT STUDY

The MedRAP pilot study was performed during the academic year 1988-1989 with a group of 12 PGY-1 residents who were recruited during orientation. The feedback from the experimental group was very positive and consistent with the feedback in subsequent years. The feedback from the original MedRAP pilot study and the senior residents suggested that the combination of a support group with a job training group format accelerated their transition to internship year and their professional development, contributing to the well-being of the PGY-1 residents.

Based on these results, the program was implemented on a full scale in July 1989 for all incoming PGY-1 residents.

LIMITATIONS OF SELF-REPORTED DATA

As with any self-reported data, the extent to which evaluations accurately reflect the program's true impact cannot be fully determined. Not all participants completed and turned in the Annual MedRAP Evaluation. Furthermore, due to survey anonymity, it is difficult to determine the number of sessions each respondent attended. Finally, while testimonies suggest that the program's return on investment (ROI) is high, substantiating objective data, such as the program's impact on reducing medical errors and increasing efficiency, is more difficult to quantify.

PROGRAM EVOLUTION

As a living program that rapidly responds to changes in needs of the residents as well as the training program, MedRAP consistently evolved based on the ongoing and continuous needs assessment conducted annually. Sessions were dropped and added through the years. For example, the session about nurse interaction was dropped after several years as the residency program improved and its demographic changed. The percentage of American graduates in the program increased and the percentage of international medical graduates (IMGs) decreased. The American graduates, accustomed to interacting with nurses in the hospitals, did not feel they were experiencing as many problems as the IMGs, and suggested that this session be dropped.

Through the years, some of the sessions were expanded based on residents' and program management feedback. For example, the QI presentation started as a one-hour presentation to all the chiefs of Internal Medicine in the different Baylor-affiliated hospitals. Over the years, the administration, the residents, and the management of the health care team perceived the QI as an important tool in improving the quality and efficiency of care. It was thus expanded to include an average of four 3- to 4-hour annual presentations for each affiliated hospital. The presentations by the senior residents were attended by the affiliated hospital administration, the health care team management, and the program directors.

CHAPTER 19:

LESSONS LEARNED AND LOOKING TO THE FUTURE

MedRAP's program has greatly evolved and benefited from the lessons learned during more than 25 years of successful program implementation. Lessons learned have been continuously incorporated into the program design. For similar programs to be successful, it is instrumental to have the following attributes:

- Secure high-level management support for the program
- Ensure that the program meets real rather than assumed needs
- Respond effectively to both participants' and management needs and goals
- Have facilitators who are familiar with organizational theory principles, medical systems and terminology, and who are effective in leading groups
- Involve faculty so they feel part of the process by:
    - Serving as facilitators (see "mixed faculty model" in Chapter 2)
    - Serving on a task force to provide feedback on program design
    - Formulating and evaluating goals and objectives
    - Testing the efficacy of the program
    - Evaluating the attainment of competencies
- Demonstrate that the program is cost-effective
- Foster a safe environment to ensure honest feedback and self-reflection

THE IMPORTANCE OF OPERATIONAL INDEPENDENCE

An effective program to improve the well-being of residents should provide a safe place for them to express their grievances. Forty-six percent of residents worry about being labeled a "troublemaker" if they complain or raise concerns about their training program. Therefore, a confidential environment provides a place where constructive change can be discussed.[1]

After 25 years of program implementation, the professional independent facilitator who had developed and implemented the program assumed other responsibilities, and junior faculty, from the same residency program, chose to run the program internally to receive some educational credit and reduce costs. After several attempts to replicate the program, it was realized that the program in its entirety can only be duplicated effectively with a facilitator who is operationally independent of the residency program and does not participate in the residents' evaluations.

Table 4 represents data from an online survey created by MedRAP's group leaders, independently and of their own volition. The survey was sent to all participants for an assessment of the program's impact. Almost 70% of respondents strongly agreed or agreed that it was important that the program be run by a facilitator who was not their faculty or evaluator.

Close to 80% of respondents strongly agreed or agreed that MedRAP sessions provided them an opportunity to give constructive feedback to the residency program.

Table 4: Online Survey Analysis of MedRAP Program Impact - Created by Residents

Variable	No. (%) of Responders	
Residency Program Type		
Internal Medicine	54	(71.1)
Internal Medicine-Pediatrics	16	(21.1)
Preliminary	6	(7.9)
Year of Training		
PGY-1	31	(40.8)
PGY-2	17	(22.4)
PGY-3	22	(28.9)
PGY-4	6	(71.9)
Important that MedRAP is run by independent facilitators, who are not faculty or evaluators		
Strongly Disagree	1	(1.4)
Disagree	7	(9.6)
Neutral	14	(19.2)
Agree	22	(30.1)
Strongly Agree	29	(39.7)
MedRAP sessions provided opportunity to give feedback		
Strongly Disagree	0	(0.0)
Disagree	4	(5.6)
Neutral	11	(15.3)
Agree	26	(36.1)
Strongly Agree	31	(43.1)

Abbreviation: PGY, Postgraduate Year.

SAFE ENVIRONMENT FACTOR (SEF)

One of the key advantages of having operationally independent MedRAP facilitators is their contribution to the Safe Environment Factor (SEF). The safe environment provided by MedRAP positively impacted residents' ability to communicate problems they were experiencing in the hospital wards, the inefficiencies they noticed in the hospital system and patient care, and challenges in the development of their own skills and competencies. The table below demonstrates how the SEF impacted the program curriculum across the board.

SKILLS/ COMPETENCIES	SAFE ENVIRONMENT FACTOR (SEF)
Organizational Skills	• Residents more likely to report their own mistakes and problems they experience with health care team functioning
Communication Skills	• Residents more likely to discuss negative feelings towards patients, families, faculty, and health care team • Residents more likely to report situational or personal issues
Quality Improvement/ Management Skills	• Residents more likely to report problems in hospital efficiency and patient care without fearing repercussions
Leadership Skills	• Residents more likely to report negative experiences with senior residents • Residents more likely to reflect on their own weaknesses as a leader
Annual Evaluation and Planning	• Residents were able to identify which components of the program worked and which did not, without worrying about communicating negative feedback to faculty who evaluate them

TRANSFERABLE COMPONENTS OF MEDRAP

MedRAP was originally developed to facilitate the transition of residents from medical school to residency. However, by providing a vision of what can be achieved in both medical education and organizational change, this book is relevant to anyone interested in improving organizational professionalism within health care, and offers strategies to maximize staff effectiveness in other areas. MedRAP is applicable to leadership of medical institutions, faculty, and program directors in medical, nursing, and allied health training programs.

The following transferable components have relevance to other health care professionals in training:

- Orientations designed for special populations and systems
- Sessions that teach the informal curriculum
- Integration of best practices in each session
- Training, which includes the development of:
  - Leadership skills
  - Organizational skills
  - Communication skills
- Quality improvement methodology to optimize patient care
- Acceleration of the flow of information to top-level management, while also engaging in collaboration with middle management

The components of the program can be modified for a range of participant requirements by utilizing specially designed needs assessments, and by individualizing the curriculum and methodology to the specific challenges and needs of each population.

In academic medicine, the program is applicable and can be tailored to the needs of:
- Residents in different specialties
- Medical students
- Fellows
- Junior medical faculty
- Nurses in residency
- Physician assistants
- Nurse practitioners

In clinical environments, some of the sessions can be adapted to the needs of:
- Practicing physicians
- Nurses
- Allied health providers

CONCLUSION

It is now widely accepted that formal wellness and well-being programs should be an integral component of physician training for the following reasons:[1]

- Programs to improve well-being and wellness are demonstrably effective.
- Residents are highly receptive to well-being curricula.
- Participation in such sessions has been correlated with higher clinician empathy.
- Well-being is associated with reduced rates of anxiety and depression among health care professionals.
- Stress management workshops have demonstrated reductions in burnout scores in health care professionals.
- Investing in well-being programs is associated with overall improvements in the delivery, efficiency, and effectiveness of care.

Programs such as MedRAP—carefully designed to be comprehensive and integrated, to prevent and reduce stress, and to promote well-being associated with burnout reduction—can make a difference for clinicians, hospitals, and medical institutions. Effective interventions can be inexpensive, and relatively small investments can produce a significant impact and lead to a large return on investment.

It is the author's hope that some of the change and innovation that positively impacted the lives of residents in the MedRAP program can benefit health care trainees in other institutions. The well-being of all health care professionals can be greatly improved by investing in their professional development and reforming their work and training environment to benefit the entire health care system, since what helps the physician, helps the patient.

WHAT HURTS THE PHYSICIAN HURTS THE PATIENT

MedRAP Facilitator Manual

Curriculum developed by Iris Mushin, M.ED., MBA

Contributing Editor, Sasha Alexander, MBA

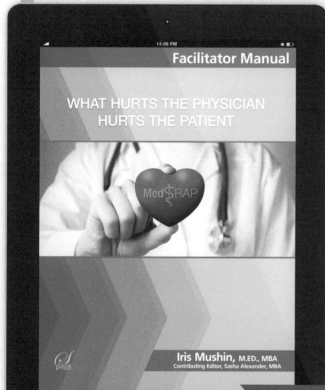

The *MedRAP Facilitator Manual*, which is available for the different topic chapters, is an e-book containing detailed and specific information on implementing and facilitating individual session topics, including facilitator guidelines and scripts for Group Leader (GL) and PGY-1 sessions. Strategies presented in the sessions are based on feedback and collective wisdom from the group leaders on best practices regarding specific challenges, as well as facilitator input, and selected approaches from leading researchers in different disciplines.

The topic sessions have been tailored to the needs of residents in Internal Medicine and Medicine Pediatrics. The information and handouts provide instructions on customizing the program for multiple settings. A sample topic chapter is provided on the following pages.

Download your e-book from any major online retailer.
E-book ISBN 978-1-944952-21-1

The MedRAP Facilitator Manual can only be used effectively in conjunction with the book, *What Hurts the Physician Hurts the Patient*. Successful implementation of MedRAP requires a thorough understanding of the program's fundamental building blocks and philosophy, carefully developed over more than two decades. Multiple strategies and tools that would lead to a program's success are presented only in the book, and the manual serves as a supplement. In addition, important information – such as instructions for conducting the Systems-Based Practice Quality Improvement — is only included in the book, not in the manual. Facilitators are strongly encouraged to thoroughly read the book in order to understand the rationale behind its design and implement it successfully.

Facilitator Manual Sample

Interacting with Patients' Families

Curriculum developed by Iris Mushin, M.Ed., MBA
Contributing editor, Sasha Alexander, MBA

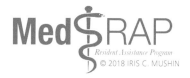

INTERACTING WITH PATIENTS' FAMILIES

Session Goal:

To provide residents with strategies, tools, and tips to effectively manage families and contribute to patient care and satisfaction.

Group Leader (GL) Session: Interacting with Patients' Families

GL SESSION OBJECTIVES

- To identify typical difficult situations postgraduate year 1 (PGY-1) residents are likely to encounter when interacting with families.
- To have GLs self-reflect on their own personal challenges when dealing with families so they can be more effective as group leaders.
- To update, revise, and tailor program materials for current needs of residents.

Feedback

(20 minutes*) *All suggested times are subject to facilitator judgment

Prior to the topic-specific discussion, the facilitator collects general feedback about GLs' rotation experiences for several reasons:

- To address the different types of problems PGY-2 and PGY-3 residents experience
- To provide GLs with the opportunity to confidentially report feedback
- To allow GLs to discuss urgent problems encountered on the wards while preserving a constructive atmosphere during PGY-1 sessions

Issues to focus on when collecting feedback:

- Strengths and weaknesses of current rotation
- Constructive feedback that could improve the rotation experience
- Collective wisdom to impart to PGY-1 residents to help them function more effectively in the rotation

Self-Reflection
(30 minutes)

These self-reflection exercises, related to the topic of discussion, help GLs to analyze problems and develop strategies to overcome difficulties they experience.

- Administer **Challenging Encounters with Families: Group Leader Questionnaire (Appendix I)** to help GLs identify situations that lead to difficult interactions.
- Ask GLs to describe a specific difficult family interaction they have encountered that is representative of situations PGY-1 residents are likely to encounter.
- Discuss and compare strategies to deal with difficult encounters.
- Ask GLs to identify families that elicit negative feelings and identify the source of these feelings (transference). Did their response to these negative feelings change through the years?
- To normalize the negative feelings residents have towards certain families and to help them facilitate discussion in the PGY-1 session, ask GLs to share some of the negative feelings they have had.

Review of Materials
(45 minutes)

Review the existing PGY-1 materials on the topic. GLs and facilitator discuss possible additions or changes to the materials that will be used in the PGY-1 sessions.

- Review **Challenging Encounters with Families: Cases for Discussion (Appendix II)** handout which has some examples of families who are generally difficult for health care professionals to handle. Determine which cases are most representative of typical situations and provide most helpful strategies. Amend the handout with GLs, developing new cases and removing irrelevant cases as needed.
  - This handout corresponds to the handout on **Challenging Encounters with Families: Managing Communication with Families (Appendix III).**
- Review **Managing Communication with Families** handout which outlines a multitude of family styles, as well as their corresponding symptoms, and offer strategies to deal with them. Ask GLs if any additional family styles need to be added that are particularly noteworthy for their hospitals, if applicable.
  - Some of the family styles are specifically discussed in **The "Challenging" Family: Cases for Discussion** and the remainder can be addressed at the end of the session or independently by the PGY-1 residents.
- Review the **Challenging Encounters with Families – Group Leader Outline (Appendix IV)** to prepare the GLs for the PGY-1 session format.

Addition of Materials
(15 minutes)

GLs suggest additional materials or exercises, relating to the topic, that they feel would be most helpful to the PGY-1 residents.

Individual Assistance
(after completion of group session)

Facilitator provides individual assistance to GLs experiencing personal or professional adjustment issues or wanting to discuss concerns about specific rotation, peers or colleagues.

Following the GL session, the facilitator reviews the feedback and suggested materials provided by the senior residents. With the GL feedback in mind, the facilitator revises the material for the PGY-1 sessions, as necessary, determining the most beneficial material to be used in the cases, handouts, and presentations. If more complex issues or ideas arise during the GL session, the facilitator continues to work directly with a few of the GLs to develop the strategies and new materials. All facilitator-determined activities and handouts will be presented during the PGY-1 sessions.

PGY-1 Sessions: Interacting with Patients' Families

PGY-1 SESSION OBJECTIVES

- To employ some basic techniques of managing and communicating with families, recognizing the basic categories of challenging families to anticipate and respond to their dynamics.
- To manage the interaction with each family category
- To tailor the communication to each family
- To set boundaries and limits in a positive way
- To prevent potential problems

General Introduction*
(5 minutes) *All suggested times are subject to facilitator judgment

Introduce group members and group leaders (GLs). Announce topic.

Feedback
(20 minutes)

Before beginning topic-specific discussion, the facilitator pauses to collect general feedback on PGY-1 residents' rotation experiences:

- Discuss present rotation and any special issues that need to be addressed regarding this rotation.
- Identify strengths and weaknesses of the rotation.
- Identify any individual difficulties that need to be dealt with privately.
- Request constructive feedback from peers and GLs that could improve the rotation experience and/or could help with any challenging situations that have been brought up.
- Facilitate communication between GLs and PGY-1 residents regarding effective strategies that have worked for them in the past.

Topic Introduction
(5 minutes)

Introduce topic and session objectives.

- Some patients' families can be difficult to handle and, thus, a great source of anger and irritation – especially for an inexperienced physician.
- These "challenging" families can refer to the conduct of a healthy family in an abnormal situation or a family with maladaptive dynamics under any circumstances.
- Either way, the common denominator between these families is their need for effective communication, which includes setting boundaries.
- While it is not possible, in one session, to identify and describe every category of challenging family you will encounter, there will be tools distributed that provide additional insight and useful strategies.

Self-Reflection
(20 minutes)

These self-reflection exercises, related to the topic of discussion, help PGY-1 residents to analyze problems and develop strategies to overcome difficulties they experience.

- Ask GLs to share with the group the types of families they find difficult to work with personally.
- Help PGY-1 residents identify the types of families they find difficult (the specific strategies for dealing with these families are addressed later in the session).

Discussion questions for PGY-1 residents:

- What type of family elicits a negative response in you?
- What type of family do you find working with most difficult?
- Are there types of families that you are more likely to encounter in certain hospitals or on specific rotations?
- Review PowerPoint presentation on **Communication with Families, Part I (Appendix V)**.

Topic Exercises, Suggested Strategies and Best Practices
(60 minutes)

These exercises facilitate experiential learning related to the session topic.

Review Cases:

The handout **Challenging Encounters with Families: Cases for Discussion (Appendix II)** has some examples of typical difficult situations residents are likely to encounter.

This handout corresponds to the handout on **Managing Communication with Families (Appendix III).** Please note that the categories of families can overlap and are not exclusive. There is not necessarily a right or wrong answer. The cases are utilized as a catalyst for PGY-1 residents to start thinking about some difficult types of situations before they have to deal with these circumstances in real life.

Case discussion flow:

- A PGY-1 reads the case
- The same PGY-1 responds with what (s)he would do
- The question raised in the case is opened up to the other PGY-1s, asking what they think or would do
- Once PGY-1s have offered their feedback, then ask the GLs what they would do
- Facilitator summarizes to wrap up case

CASE A:

You are a PGY-I resident on the Renal Service. One of your patients, Jack, is a 29-year-old who has recently been admitted with chronic renal failure. He is diabetic and hypertensive. He has a Quinton catheter, has been on Hemodialysis for several days, and is scheduled to have an insertion of an Access Graft in a few days.

His wife always has many, many questions and talking to her consumes a great deal of your time. It is difficult for you to leave their room because the family members always have one more question to ask. They are forever asking about the significance of tiny changes, such as variations in potassium levels, and frequently ask questions that you can't really answer, like, "Will he be able to receive a kidney transplant soon?" They request that the nurse call you for every electrolyte check and want you to OK each medication dose personally, even though he has been on the same medications for three days. Throughout the day, you receive many phone calls from different concerned relatives.

How would you manage this family?

Follow-up discussion and suggested strategies for the facilitator

1. *Why is the family acting this way?*
2. *Is it possible something else is motivating this behavior?*
3. *Is there a way to set time boundaries in a positive way?*

Tips and Tools

- Have the family appoint a spokesperson; one cannot spend the entire day answering calls from different family members, often answering the same questions.

- Initially, give them a full explanation and background; however, some families will always want more information or more of the physician's time. Learning to set boundaries is essential. Examples of setting boundaries:
  - Set time for the meeting
  - Limit time of meeting
  - Instruct family to write down questions and discuss the most important ones at the meeting
- Such behaviors can be a sign of families feeling out of control. Giving them a role to help the health care team might be helpful (for example, watching vital signs or taking temperature).
- There is a limit to physicians' stamina. It is important to learn to set limits as early as possible, and in a positive way. It is not in the best interest of physicians or patients that health care professionals burn out.
- Some families are needy and get a secondary gain from interacting with the physician. The more they receive, the more they want. Setting appropriate expectations can assist.

CASE B:

Mrs. Gonzales is the 57-year-old matriarch of a large family and was admitted to your service 4 days ago for increased shortness of breath. She is a pack-a-day smoker. She underwent a needle biopsy of a large right upper lobe mass.

The family members, very visible at the bedside, anxiously await the results of the fine needle biopsy. Each time you enter the room, they ask how their mother is doing and what you think the biopsy will show. They repeatedly tell you what a wonderful doctor you are and that they are sure you will make their mother better.

You have just walked into the room when one of the daughters hands you a wrapped box and says, "It is just a small token of our appreciation; we know that with a doctor like you, Mother is going to be just fine."

How would you handle this situation?

Follow-up discussion and suggested strategies for the facilitator

1. *Which style best describes the family in this case?*
2. *What could be motivating the family to present a gift to the physician?*
3. *Is it appropriate to accept gifts from patients? If yes, in which situations? What can be done with this gift without hurting the family's feelings?*

*(Refer to strategies for Anxiety-Ridden Families in the **Managing Communication with Families** handout.)*

- Discuss strategies presented in the handout
- In terms of handling the gift (to avoid bargaining)
  - Set the family's expectations appropriately and remind them that the biopsy could come back positive;
  - It may be necessary to decline acceptance of the gift graciously; or
  - In order to stay culturally sensitive, explain to the family that the entire health care team works together and the gift will be shared appropriately.

CASE C:

You are a first-year resident on the Hem/Onc service. One of your patients is an 18-year-old girl who came from out of town with her parents and has been diagnosed with Acute Leukemia.

You round twice daily with patients on this service. You visited the patient in the morning for several minutes and told the worried mother that you will see her later that afternoon, around 5:00 pm to discuss the plans and answer questions. Due to an emergency, you arrive forty-five minutes late to the conference with the family.

As you walk into the room, the parents appear angry and hostile. The mother tells you: "We have been waiting for you for almost two hours. You are always late; we are unhappy with the care our daughter has been getting. We are very disappointed with the hospital. Nobody here seems to really care about patients."

How would you respond to the parents?

Follow-up discussion and suggested strategies for the facilitator

1. *Why is the family behaving this way?*
2. *What can be done to defuse the situation?*

[Review the **Communication with Families, Part II (Appendix V)** PowerPoint presentation for suggested strategies] [1-3]

- Discuss using empathy: It is not possible to feel everything the family is feeling. An empathic listener identifies the emotion in the person speaking, identifies the cause of the emotion, and responds in a way that makes a connection between the two. For example: "You are very upset because you don't think the doctors are spending enough time with your son"; "You seem to be worried because you are not sure of the prognosis and treatment option."
- Discuss the Inquiry Technique: In this case study, the mother says that she is very unhappy with the hospital. She could be unhappy with the nurses, the attending

physician, or even you – and it is better to find out before she complains to the attending physician. People are often reluctant to express their thoughts and confront directly, but they may redirect their anger. It is better to give them permission to express their frustrations in order to address the complaints before they act.

- At times, people do not proactively and effectively communicate their concerns about problems they experience in order to avoid confrontation. The trick is constructively addressing the issues early enough, before problems escalate.
- These techniques could also be used in effectively managing teams.

CASE D:

A patient has just told you confidentially that he has had an affair while out of town. His wife also happens to be your patient. Since his return, he has had sexual relations with her.

Now he has a penile discharge and he asks you to treat them both with antibiotics for his supposed Urinary Tract Infection. He suggests that you recommend she receive prophylactic antibiotics.

How would you respond?

Follow-up discussion and suggested strategies for the facilitator

1. *Is it ethical or legal to do what the patient has requested?*
2. *What are the options for handling this situation?*

- Discuss ethical conduct and setting boundaries appropriately.
- Advise the patient ahead of time that there is a limit to a physician's ability to keep secrets.
- A physician should not be lying to his patient.
- One way to help is offering to facilitate communication.
- Raise the question about whether it is possible that the wife contracted the infection and gave it to her husband.

CASE E:

Mr. Evans is a 66-year-old man who was transferred to your service from the Neuro ICU. He is 3 months S/P cardiac arrest at home with second degree severe anoxic encephalopathy, requiring intubation, ventilator support and intensive nursing care for decubitus ulcers.

His wife and daughter, as well as his son, who had not seen him in 15 years, are always at his bedside. They constantly harass the nursing staff and you about multiple small details of their father's care. They refuse to discuss code status and get angry when the subject is brought up. You have overheard the son say, "These doctors are going to be in trouble if Dad does not get better soon."

How would you handle this situation?

Follow-up discussion and suggested strategies for the facilitator

1. *Why is this family acting in this manner?*
2. *What are some of the emotions the family is currently experiencing?*

(Refer to strategies for Guilt-Ridden Families in the **Managing Communication with Families** handout.)

- The family members are guilt-ridden because they have not seen the father in 15 years. Their regrets are manifested in projected anger towards the health care professional, and need to be redirected.
- Help them to separate their guilt and regrets from misplaced anger. They cannot change the situation or the prognosis, and need to consider what is in the father's best interest.
- Malpractice cases often come from these types of situations.
- DOCUMENT EVERYTHING!

Conclusion
(10 minutes)

Summarize the best practices and strategies identified relating to the topic.

- Try to think systematically about the families you encounter.
- If you are able to categorize them and recognize similarities to families you previously encountered, you can utilize strategies you found to be effective with this particular family type.
- These techniques can be helpful with co-workers, health care team members, and even in your personal lives – not just with patients.

Individual Assistance
(after group session completion)

Facilitator provides individual assistance to residents experiencing personal or professional adjustment issues.

Challenging Encounters with Families: Group Leader Questionnaire

What type of families do you have difficulties working with?

_____

_____

_____

_____

Are there specific families that elicit uncomfortable or negative responses in you? What is the cause of your uncomfortable or negative response?

_____

_____

_____

_____

What are the most difficult challenges you face when working with families?

_____

_____

_____

_____

Are there particular challenges in dealing with families in different affiliated hospitals or services?

_____

_____

_____

_____

Is there any particular difficult situation you wish you would have handled differently? Please describe in detail (to be used as case studies for PGY-1 residents).

_____

_____

_____

_____

Do you have any additional tips or suggestions for PGY-1 residents?

_____

_____

_____

_____

Challenging Encounters with Families: Cases for Discussion

CASE A:

You are a PGY-I resident on the Renal Service. One of your patients, Jack, is a 29-year-old who has recently been admitted with chronic renal failure. He is diabetic and hypertensive. He has a Quinton catheter, has been on Hemodialysis for several days, and is scheduled to have an insertion of an Access Graft in a few days.

His wife always has many, many questions and talking to her consumes a great deal of your time. It is difficult for you to leave their room because the family members always have one more question to ask. They are forever asking about the significance of tiny changes, such as variations in potassium levels, and frequently ask questions that you can't really answer, like, "Will he be able to receive a kidney transplant soon?" They request that the nurse call you for every electrolyte check and want you to OK each medication dose personally, even though he has been on the same medications for three days. Throughout the day, you receive many phone calls from different concerned relatives.

How would you manage this family?

CASE B:

Mrs. Gonzales is the 57-year-old matriarch of a large family and was admitted to your service 4 days ago for increased shortness of breath. She is a pack-a-day smoker. She underwent a needle biopsy of a large right upper lobe mass.

The family members, very visible at the bedside, anxiously await the results of the fine needle biopsy. Each time you enter the room, they ask how their mother is doing and what you think the biopsy will show. They repeatedly tell you what a wonderful doctor you, are and that they are sure you will make their mother better.

You have just walked into the room when one of the daughters hands you a wrapped box and says, "It is just a small token of our appreciation; we know that with a doctor like you, Mother is going to be just fine."

How would you handle this situation?

CASE C:

You are a first-year resident on the Hem/Onc service. One of your patients is an 18-year-old girl who came from out of town with her parents and has been diagnosed with Acute Leukemia.

You round twice daily with patients on this service. You visited the patient in the morning for several minutes and told the worried mother that you will see her later that afternoon, around 5:00 pm to discuss the plans and answer questions. Due to an emergency, you arrive forty-five minutes late to the conference with the family.

As you walk into the room, the parents appear angry and hostile. The mother tells you: "We have been waiting for you for almost two hours. You are always late; we are unhappy with the care our daughter has been getting. We are very disappointed with the hospital. Nobody here seems to really care about patients."

How would you respond to the parents?

CASE D:

A patient has just told you confidentially that he has had an affair while out of town. His wife also happens to be your patient. Since his return, he has had sexual relations with her.

Now he has a penile discharge and he asks you to treat them both with antibiotics for his supposed Urinary Tract Infection. He suggests that you recommend she receive prophylactic antibiotics.

How would you respond?

CASE E:

Mr. Evans is a 66-year-old man who was transferred to your service from the Neuro ICU. He is 3 months S/P cardiac arrest at home with second degree severe anoxic encephalopathy, requiring intubation, ventilator support and intensive nursing care for decubitus ulcers.

His wife and daughter, as well as his son, who had not seen him in 15 years, are always at his bedside. They constantly harass the nursing staff and you about multiple small details of their father's care. They refuse to discuss code status and get angry when the subject is brought up. You have overheard the son say, "These doctors are going to be in trouble if Dad does not get better soon."

How would you handle this situation?

Challenging Encounters with Families: Managing Communication with Families*

Please note:

- The styles offer broad definitions and characteristics.
- Styles are non-exclusive. Families can often exhibit a multitude of styles simultaneously.
- The symptoms observed may be an exacerbated version of the family's true style due to the stress caused by the circumstances.

STYLE	SYMPTOMS	STRATEGIES
Disorganized	Lacking structure, having no goals, no major persons of authority, much confusion, poor communication, seeks dependence upon institutions and authority figures outside the family.	When interviewing, provide structure; take control. Define a spokesperson for the group. Simplify your approach/management plan to make it easier for the patient and family to comply. Written instructions are vital. Define expectations for the hospitalization.
Anxiety-Ridden	Remains constantly by patient. Tries to solicit information from other sources. Asks for constant reassurance, misinterprets information. Feels that telling the doctor what a good doctor he is will magically affect the outcome.	Start preparing the family early. Structure communication. Say the same thing to all members. Keep professional distance. Be careful of extra positive reinforcement. Try to avoid accepting gifts. Ask to please show gratitude to entire department. Set time for daily conferences.

---

* Based on *Physician stress: a handbook for coping.*[4]

Enmeshed	Rarely leaves patient bedside. Angered when restricted from seeing patient. Inhibits patient from having one-to-one relations with doctor. Many times, doctor is portrayed in an unfavorable light. Serves as clearinghouse for medical information; hides diagnosis from patient.	Take control while at the same time acknowledging that the family member is trying to care for the patient. Give family members small tasks so they feel less helpless. Prevention is key – set realistic expectations from the beginning.
Dependent	Unending need for contact and support. Insecure. Perceive the doctor as an inexhaustible provider. Has an insatiable need for constant contact.	Set clear, firm limits on the role and availability of staff. Avoid reacting with aversion and avoidance. Provide *early* social service or psychiatric referral.
Decompensated	Family insists that the patient is deteriorating, though symptoms are chronic. Family members grow tired of taking care of patient themselves.	Offer help; use social workers to come up with options re: placement / transportation / respite care.
Intimidating or Entitled	Pretend to know vast amount of medical information. Demand certain types of medications and treatments, questioning doctor's judgment. Allude to malpractice, indicating to the doctor that they are influential in the community and will ruin his/her reputation. Being rude to doctor. Want control over doctor.	Clear contract should be established with patient (bypass family, if possible). Try to educate and involve family members in decision-making, but recognize that it is okay to set boundaries. Keep family informed of any adverse consequences. Use disarming technique. If the above measures fail, consider involving the higher authorities / consulting Ethics.

Denying	Uses denial to cope with stress. Inattentive to instructions which could lead to noncompliance. Avoids dealing with personal emotions.	Acknowledge the difficulty of having a sick family member. Avoid emotionality; provide reading material on the illness. Encourage the family to speak with other families in similar circumstances.
Uncooperative or Abusive	Unconcerned about family member. Resistant to speaking with the doctor and carrying out his or her recommendations. Leaves the patient in the hospital to recover.	Use contractual approach. Appeal to their conscience. Use social workers to come up with options re: placement / transportation / respite care. Try to determine family's motivation and limitations. Involve APS if necessary.
Irrational or Unrealistic	Family members make unreasonable requests such as prescribing high doses of vitamins or demanding inpatient consultations for issues that could be handled as outpatient.	Try to find out what is motivating the request(s). It is okay to 'bargain' as long as you 'do no harm' (e.g. prescribe a multivitamin instead).
Expecting Miracles	Family circumvents discussion of important matters e.g. code status / direction of care, stating that the patient's health is 'in God's hands.'	Work within the family's belief system, involve a chaplain if possible. For instance, you can reframe the code issue as follows: "The life support we are providing for your loved one is very artificial and outside of God's realm; perhaps we should focus on comfort, withdraw the artificial support and let God determine the outcome."
Guilt-Ridden	Unable to decide plans for aging parent. Inability to control anger. Project guilt onto other persons (doctor). Malpractice suits; very demanding of attention.	Alleviate guilt by defining realistic expectations; be consistent and brief. Document *everything*! Emphasize that decision must be made, because situation will NOT change.

Challenging Encounters with Families: Group Leader Outline

I. **Group members introduction and collection of ongoing feedback**

II. **Identification of families that are difficult to work with and/or elicit negative responses**

   a. Group Leaders describe type of families they find difficult to work with (strategies are discussed later in session)

      i. GL descriptions set the tone and give permission to PGY-1 residents to discuss negative feelings

      ii. The goal is to show the PGY-1 residents that it is normal to feel frustrated with patient families. Ultimately, it is how you manage those feelings that counts (tools are provided later in session)

   b. PGY-1 residents describe type of families they find difficult to work with

III. **PowerPoint Presentation on Communication with Families Part I**

IV. **Discussion of The Difficult Family cases (Appendix II) and Identification of Styles (Appendix III)**

   a. A PGY-1 resident reads and discusses his/her responses to cases

      i. Other PGY-1 residents provide feedback

      ii. GLs provide feedback

   b. Review strategies in **PowerPoint Presentation on Communication with Families Part II**, following Case C discussion

Challenging Encounters with Families: PowerPoint Presentations

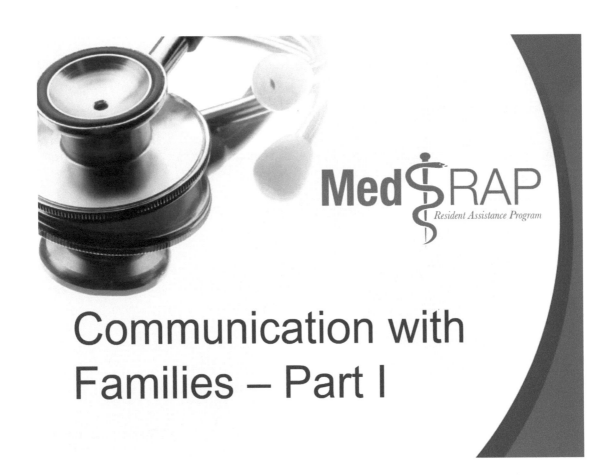

Communication with Families – Part I

"Difficult" Families

- Some families are difficult for health care professionals to manage

- Taking care of a patient with a "difficult" family can be a great source of anger and irritation

"Difficult" Families

- "Difficult" family can refer to:
  - Conduct of a healthy family in an abnormal situation
  - Family with maladaptive dynamics under any circumstances

- The common denominator:
  - Family's need for *effective communication* by physician

Communication is not just an art

…It's also a science

Cognitive skill
Learned intellectual process

Medical Communication

Possible to teach these skills

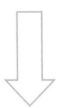

If you break down
communication into its
components

False Assumptions

- If I provide high quality care…

- If I follow established standard practices in my specialty…

      …I will NOT be sued

Communication Breakdown

Many malpractice depositions cite communication breakdowns between physicians and their patients or patients' families

When Faced With a Bad Outcome

Patients and families are likely to reflect on whether the physician:

- Was caring and compassionate

- Invested the needed time in the patient's management

Satisfied patients and families are more likely to forgive

Session Goals

- Learn to recognize basic categories of "difficult" families so you are not caught off guard by their dynamics

- Learn to employ some basic techniques to manage and communicate with them

PowerPoint Presentation on Communication with Families Part II

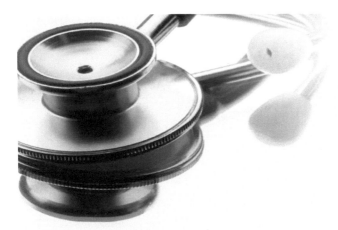

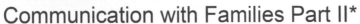
Communication with Families Part II*

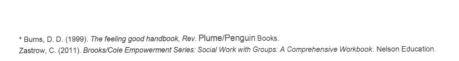
* Burns, D. D. (1999). *The feeling good handbook, Rev.* Plume/Penguin Books.
Zastrow, C. (2011). *Brooks/Cole Empowerment Series: Social Work with Groups: A Comprehensive Workbook.* Nelson Education.

Strategies

- The Disarming Technique

- Empathy
  - Thought empathy
  - Feeling empathy

- Inquiry

Disarming Technique

Find some truth in what the other person is saying, even if it seems unfair and unreasonable

Disarming Technique

- Usually when you agree with the other person, s/he will then stop arguing

- Regardless of how wrong the criticism might seem, find some grain of truth in it

Disarming Technique

- Do not be defensive. When you resist the urge to defend yourself and instead agree with the other person, you will often, surprisingly, end up finding an effective resolution

- S/he will usually feel then much more open to your point of view

Disarming Technique

- An effective tool when you feel criticized and attacked

- Takes "the wind" out of the other person's sails and has a calming effect

Empathy

Put yourself in the other person's shoes and try to see the world through his or her eyes

- **Thought empathy**

  Paraphrase the other person's words

- **Feeling empathy**

  Acknowledge how s/he might be feeling

Inquiry

Gently ask probing questions to discover the other person's thoughts and feelings

Inquiry

Get the other person to "lay his cards on the table" so you can deal with the problem and know where you stand

REFERENCES

CHAPTER 1

1. Shanafelt, T. D., & Noseworthy, J. H. (2017, January). Executive leadership and physician well-being: nine organizational strategies to promote engagement and reduce burnout. In *Mayo Clinic Proceedings* (Vol. 92, No. 1, pp. 129-146). Elsevier.

2. Bodenheimer, T., & Sinsky, C. (2014). From triple to quadruple aim: care of the patient requires care of the provider. *The Annals of Family Medicine,12*(6), 573-576.

3. Shanafelt, T. D., Dyrbye, L. N., & West, C. P. (2017). Addressing Physician Burnout: The Way Forward. *Jama,317*(9), 901-902.

4. Wallace, J. E., Lemaire, J. B., & Ghali, W. A. (2009). Physician wellness: a missing quality indicator. *The Lancet,374*(9702), 1714-1721.

5. Dunn, P. M., Arnetz, B. B., Christensen, J. F., & Homer, L. (2007). Meeting the imperative to improve physician well-being: assessment of an innovative program. *Journal of general internal medicine,22*(11), 1544-1552.

6. Spinelli, W. M. (2013, December). The phantom limb of the triple aim. In *Mayo Clinic Proceedings* (Vol. 88, No. 12, pp. 1356-1357). Elsevier.

7. Shanafelt, T. D., Boone, S., Tan, L., Dyrbye, L. N., Sotile, W., Satele, D., ... & Oreskovich, M. R. (2012). Burnout and satisfaction with work-life balance among US physicians relative to the general US population. *Archives of internal medicine,172*(18), 1377-1385.

8. Firth-Cozens, J. (2001). Interventions to improve physicians' well-being and patient care. *Social science & medicine,52*(2), 215-222.

9. Sargent, M. C., Sotile, W., Sotile, M. O., Rubash, H., & Barrack, R. L. (2004). Stress and coping among orthopaedic surgery residents and faculty. *The Journal of Bone & Joint Surgery, 86*(7), 1579-1586.

10. Firth-Cozens, J. (1998). Individual and organizational predictors of depression in general practitioners. *British Journal of General Practice, 48*(435), 1647-1651.

11. Frank, E., & Dingle, A. D. (1999). Self-reported depression and suicide attempts among US women physicians. *American Journal of Psychiatry, 156*(12), 1887-1894.

12. Graham, J., Albery, I. P., Ramirez, A. J., & Richards, M. A. (2001). How hospital consultants cope with stress at work: implications for their mental health. *Stress and Health, 17*(2), 85-89.

13. Dyrbye, L. N., Thomas, M. R., Massie, F. S., Power, D. V., Eacker, A., Harper, W., & Shanafelt, T. D. (2008). Burnout and suicidal ideation among US medical students. *Annals of Internal Medicine, 149*(5), 334-341.

14. van der Heijden, F., Dillingh, G., Bakker, A., & Prins, J. (2008). Suicidal thoughts among medical residents with burnout. *Archives of Suicide Research, 12*(4), 344-346.

15. Goldman, M. L., Shah, R. N., & Bernstein, C. A. (2015). Depression and suicide among physician trainees: recommendations for a national response. *JAMA psychiatry,72*(5), 411-412.

16. Shanafelt, T., & Dyrbye, L. (2012). Oncologist burnout: causes, consequences, and responses. *Journal of Clinical Oncology,30*(11), 1235-1241.

17. Williams, E. S., Manwell, L. B., Konrad, T. R., & Linzer, M. (2007). The relationship of organizational culture, stress, satisfaction, and burnout with physician-reported error and suboptimal patient care: results from the MEMO study. *Health care management review,32*(3), 203-212.

18. Shanafelt, T. D., Bradley, K. A., Wipf, J. E., & Back, A. L. (2002). Burnout and self-reported patient care in an internal medicine residency program. *Annals of internal medicine,136*(5), 358-367.

19. Bodenheimer, T. S., & Smith, M. D. (2013). Primary care: proposed solutions to the physician shortage without training more physicians. *Health Affairs,32*(11), 1881-1886.

20. Coffey, D. S., P. Cuff, K. Eliot, E. Goldblatt, C. Grus, S. Kishore, M. Mancini, R. Valachovic, P. H. Walker. 2017. A multifaceted systems approach to addressing stress within health professions education and beyond. National Academy of Medicine, Washington, DC. https://nam.edu/wp-content/uploads/2017/01/AMultifaceted-Systems-Approach-to-AddressingStress-within-Health-Professions-Education-andBeyond.pdf

21. Shanafelt, T. D., Gorringe, G., Menaker, R., Storz, K. A., Reeves, D., Buskirk, S. J., ... & Swensen, S. J. (2015, April). Impact of organizational leadership on physician burnout and satisfaction. In *Mayo Clinic Proceedings* (Vol. 90, No. 4, pp. 432-440). Elsevier.

22. Bell, H. (2013). The burnout busters: how three Mayo Clinic physicians became experts on physician well-being. *Minnesota Medicine.* 96:11 2013 Nov pg 14-8.

23. Lefebvre, D. C. (2012). Perspective: resident physician wellness: a new hope. *Academic medicine,87*(5), 598-602.

24. IsHak, W. W., Lederer, S., Mandili, C., Nikravesh, R., Seligman, L., Vasa, M., & Bernstein, C. A. (2009). Burnout during residency training: a literature review. *Journal of Graduate Medical Education, 1*(2), 236-242.

25. Teo, A. R., Harleman, E., O'Sullivan, P. S., & Maa, J. (2011). The key role of a transition course in preparing medical students for internship. *Academic medicine: journal of the Association of American Medical Colleges,86*(7), 860.

26. Andrew, L. B., & Brenner, B. E. (2015). Physician suicide. *Medscape Drugs & Diseases.*

27. Goitein, L., Shanafelt, T. D., Wipf, J. E., Slatore, C. G., & Back, A. L. (2005). The effects of work-hour limitations on resident well-being, patient care, and education in an internal medicine residency program. *Archives of Internal Medicine, 165*(22), 2601-2606.

28. Goehring, C., Gallacchi, M. B., Kunzi, B., & Bovier, P. (2005). Psychosocial and professional characteristics of burnout in Swiss primary care practitioners: A cross-sectional survey. *Swiss Medical Weekly, 135*(7-8), 101-108.

29. Panagopoulou, E., Montgomery, A., & Benos, A. (2006). Burnout in internal medicine physicians: Differences between residents and specialists. *European Journal of Internal Medicine, 17*(3), 195-200.

30. Renzi, C., Tabolli, S., Ianni, A., Di Pietro, C., & Puddu, P. (2005). Burnout and job satisfaction comparing health care staff of a dermatological hospital and a general hospital. *Journal of the European Academy of Dermatology and Venereology, 19*(2), 153-157.

31. Fahrenkopf, A. M., Sectish, T. C., Barger, L. K., Sharek, P. J., Lewin, D., Chiang, V. W., & Landrigan, C. P. (2008). Rates of medication errors among depressed and burnt out residents: prospective cohort study. *BMJ, 336*(7642), 488-491.

32. Ripp, J., Fallar, R., Babyatsky, M., David, R., Reich, L., & Korenstein, D. (2010). Prevalence of resident burnout at the start of training. *Teaching and Learning in Medicine, 22*(3), 172-175.

33. IsHak, W. W., Lederer, S., Mandili, C., Nikravesh, R., Seligman, L., Vasa, M., ... & Bernstein, C. A. (2009). Burnout during residency training: a literature review.*Journal of graduate medical education,1*(2), 236-242.

34. Fnais, N., Soobiah, C., Chen, M. H., Lillie, E., Perrier, L., Tashkhandi, M., ... & Tricco, A. C. (2014). Harassment and discrimination in medical training: a systematic review and meta-analysis.*Academic Medicine,89*(5), 817-827.

35. Chen, P. W. (2012). The bullying culture of medical school.*The New York Times.*

36. Shanafelt, T. D. (2009). Enhancing meaning in work: a prescription for preventing physician burnout and promoting patient-centered care.*Jama,302*(12), 1338-1340.

37. Shanafelt, T. D., Sloan, J. A., & Habermann, T. M. (2003). The well-being of physicians.*The American journal of medicine,114*(6), 513-519.

38. West, C. P., Huschka, M. M., Novotny, P. J., Sloan, J. A., Kolars, J. C., Habermann, T. M., & Shanafelt, T. D. (2006). Association of perceived medical errors with resident distress and empathy: a prospective longitudinal study.*Jama,296*(9), 1071-1078.

39. Frei, E., Stamm, M., & Buddeberg-Fischer, B. (2010). Mentoring programs for medical students-a review of the PubMed literature 2000-2008.*BMC medical education,10*(1), 32.

40. Eckleberry-Hunt, J., Van Dyke, A., Lick, D., & Tucciarone, J. (2009). Changing the conversation from burnout to wellness: physician well-being in residency training programs. *Journal of Graduate Medical Education, 1*(2), 225-230.

41. Accreditation Council for Graduate Medical Education. Common program requirements. Available at: http://www.acgme.org/outcome/comp/compCPRL.asp. Accessed November 12, 2009.

42. Rosen, I. M., Gimotty, P. A., Shea, J. A., & Bellini, L. M. (2006). Evolution of sleep quantity, sleep deprivation, mood disturbances, empathy, and burnout among interns. *Academic Medicine, 81*(1), 82-85.

43. Mushin, I. C., Matteson, M. T., & Lynch, E. C. (1993). Developing a resident assistance program: beyond the support group model.*Archives of internal medicine,153*(6), 729-733.

44. Angus, S., Vu, T. R., Halvorsen, A. J., Aiyer, M., McKown, K., Chmielewski, A. F., & McDonald, F. S. (2014). What skills should new internal medicine interns have in July? A national survey of internal medicine residency program directors.*Academic Medicine,89*(3), 432-435.

45. Dyrbye, L. N., West, C. P., Satele, D., Boone, S., Tan, L., Sloan, J., & Shanafelt, T. D. (2014). Burnout among US medical students, residents, and early career physicians relative to the general US population.*Academic Medicine,89*(3), 443-451.

46. Kinkhabwala, P., Vanessa, W., Halvorsen III, O. M. S., & Escobar, D. O. (2017). Addressing Burnout, Depression, and Suicidal Ideation in the Osteopathic Profession.

47. West, C. P., Dyrbye, L. N., Erwin, P. J., & Shanafelt, T. D. (2016). Interventions to prevent and reduce physician burnout: a systematic review and meta-analysis.*The Lancet,388*(10057), 2272-2281.

48. Goebert, D., Thompson, D., Takeshita, J., Beach, C., Bryson, P., Ephgrave, K., ... & Tate, J. (2009). Depressive symptoms in medical students and residents: a multischool study. *Academic Medicine*, *84*(2), 236-241.

49. Shanafelt, T. D., West, C. P., Sloan, J. A., Novotny, P. J., Poland, G. A., Menaker, R., ... & Dyrbye, L. N. (2009). Career fit and burnout among academic faculty. *Archives of Internal Medicine*, *169*(10), 990-995.

50. Noseworthy, J., Madara, J., & Cosgrove, D. (2017). Physician burnout is a public health crisis: a message to our fellow health care CEOs.

51. Grus, C., & Kishore, S. P. (2017). A Multifaceted Systems Approach to Addressing Stress Within Health Professions Education and Beyond.

52. Weber, D. O. (August 27, 2013). Battling Physician Burnout, Part 2: To thrive, health care organizations will have to help physicians heal themselves. Accessed on 10-4-2017 from http://www.hhnmag.com/articles/5665-battling-physician-burnout-part-2

53. Krasner, M. S., Epstein, R. M., Beckman, H., Suchman, A. L., Chapman, B., Mooney, C. J., & Quill, T. E. (2009). Association of an educational program in mindful communication with burnout, empathy, and attitudes among primary care physicians. *Jama*, *302*(12), 1284-1293.

54. Slavin, S. J., Schindler, D. L., & Chibnall, J. T. (2014). Medical student mental health 3.0: improving student wellness through curricular changes. *Academic Medicine*, *89*(4), 573.

CHAPTER 2

1. Shanafelt, T. D., & Noseworthy, J. H. (2017, January). Executive leadership and physician well-being: nine organizational strategies to promote engagement and reduce burnout. In *Mayo Clinic Proceedings* (Vol. 92, No. 1, pp. 129-146). Elsevier.

2. Swensen, S., & Shanafelt, T. (2016). Physician-Organization Collaboration Reduces Physician Burnout and Promotes Engagement: The Mayo Clinic Experience. *Journal of Healthcare Management*, *61*(2), 105-127.

3. Eckleberry-Hunt, J., Van Dyke, A., Lick, D., & Tucciarone, J. (2009). Changing the conversation from burnout to wellness: physician well-being in residency training programs. *Journal of graduate medical education*, *1*(2), 225-230.

4. A Program to Create Balance in the Lives of our Residents. (n.d.). Retrieved October 05, 2017, from https://med.stanford.edu/gensurg/education/BIL.html

5. Mindful Practice. (n.d.). Retrieved October 05, 2017, from https://www.urmc.rochester.edu/family-medicine/mindful-practice.aspx

6. Resident Well-Being. (n.d.). Retrieved October 05, 2017, from http://psychresidency.ucsd.edu/apply/Pages/support.aspx

7. Saini, S. (n.d.). Resident Wellness. Retrieved October 05, 2017, from https://www.uab.edu/medicine/imresidency/resident-life/resident-wellness

8. Internal Medicine Residency Program. (2017, January 24). Retrieved October 05, 2017, from https://www.med.unc.edu/medicine/education/residency/residents/resident-wellness

9. (n.d.). Retrieved October 05, 2017, from https://smhs.gwu.edu/psychiatry/education-training/residency/wellness

10. Henry, T. A. (April 13, 2016). Preventing burnout in residency programs: Mayo Clinic's unique approach. *AMA Wire*. Accessed on 10-5-17 at https://wire.ama-assn.org/education/preventing-burn-out-residency-programs-mayo-clinics-unique-approach

11. Krasner MS, Epstein RM, Beckman H, Suchman AL, Chapman B, Mooney CJ, et al. Association of an Educational Program in Mindful Communication with Burnout, Empathy and Attitudes Among Primary Care Physicians. *JAMA* 2009; 302 (12):1284-93.

12. Satterfield JM, Becerra C. Developmental Challenges, Stressors, and Coping in Medical Residents: A Qualitative Analysis of Support Groups. *Med Educ* 2010; 44 (9):908-16.

13. Dabrow S, Russell S, Ackley K, Anderson E, Fabri PJ. Combating the Stress of Residency: One School's Approach. *Acad Med* 2006; 81 (5):436-9.

14. McCray LW, Cronholm PF, Bogner HR, Gallo JJ, Neill RA. Resident Physician Burnout: Is There Hope? *Fam Med* 2008; 40 (9):626-32.

15. Klein EJ, Marcuse EK, Jackson JC, Watkins S, Hudgins L. The Pediatric Intern Retreat: 20-year Evolution of a Continuing Investment. *Acad Med* 2000; 75 (8):853-7.

16. Devens M, Hasnain M, Dudkiewicz B, Connell KJ. Facilitating Resident Well-being: A Pilot Intervention to Address Stress and Teamwork Issues on an Inpatient Service. *Fam Med* 2012; 44 (4):265-8.

17. Klein EJ, Marcuse EK, Jackson JC, Watkins S, Hudgins L. The Pediatric Intern Retreat: 20-year Evolution of a Continuing Investment. *Acad Med* 2000; 75 (8):853-7.

18. Goldstein EA, Maestas RR, Fryer-Edwards K, Wenrich MD, Oelschlager AMA, Baernstein A, et al. Professionalism in Medical Education: An Institutional Challenge. *Acad Med* 2006; 81 (10):871-6.

19. Rousseau A, Saucier D, Côté L. Introduction to Core Competencies in Residency: A Description of an Intensive, Integrated, Multispecialty Teaching Program. *Acad Med* 2007; 82 (6):563-8.

20. Suchman AL, Williamson PR, Litzelman DK, Frankel RM, Mossbarger DL, Inui TS; and Relationship-centered Care Initiative Discovery Team. Toward an Informal Curriculum that Teaches Professionalism: Transforming the Social Environment of a Medical School. *J Gen Intern Med* 2004; 19:501-4.

21. Mosser G, Frisch KK, Skarda PK, Gertner E. Addressing the Challenges in Quality Improvement. *Am J Med* 2009; 122 (5):487-91.

22. Ogrinc G, Headrick LA, Morrison LJ, Foster T. Teaching and Assessing Resident Competence in Practice-based Learning and Improvement. *J Gen Intern Med* 2004; 19:496-500.

23. Mladenovic J, Bush R, Frohna J. Internal Medicine's Educational Interventions Project: Improving Health Care and Learning. *Am J Med* 2009; 122 (4):398-404.

24. Djuricich AM, Ciccarelli M, Swigonski NL. A Continuous Quality Improvement Curriculum for Residents: Addressing Core Competency, Improving Systems. *Acad Med* 2004; 79 (10 Suppl):S65-S67.

25. Weingart SN, Tess A, Driver J, Aronson MD, Sands K. Creating a Quality Improvement Elective for Medical House Officers. *J Gen Intern Med* 2004; 19:861-7.

26. Patow CA, Karpovich K, Riesenberg LA, Jaeger J, Rosenfeld JC, Wittenbreer M, et al. Residents' Engagement in Quality Improvement: A Systematic Review of the Literature. *Acad Med* 2009; 84 (12):1757-64.

27. Oyler J, Vinci L, Arora V, Johnson J. Teaching Internal Medicine Residents Quality Improvement Techniques using the ABIM's Practice Improvement Modules. *J Gen Intern Med* 2008; 23 (7):927-30. doi: 10.1007/s11606-008-0549-5.

CHAPTER 3

1. Shanafelt, T. D. (2009). Enhancing meaning in work: a prescription for preventing physician burnout and promoting patient-centered care.*Jama*,*302*(12), 1338-1340.

2. Shanafelt, T. D., Bradley, K. A., Wipf, J. F., & Back, A. L. (2002). Burnout and self-reported patient care in an internal medicine residency program.*Annals of internal medicine*,*136*(5), 358-367.

3. Kassam, A., Horton, J., Shoimer, I., & Patten, S. (2015). Predictors of well-being in resident physicians: a descriptive and psychometric study.*Journal of graduate medical education*,*7*(1), 70-74.

4. Bell, H. (2013). The burnout busters: how three Mayo Clinic physicians became experts on physician well-being. *Minnesota Medicine*. 96:11 2013 Nov pg 14-8.

5. Ahmed N, Devitt KS, Keshet I, et al. A Systematic Review of the Effects of Resident Duty Hour Restrictions in Surgery: Impact on Resident Wellness, Training, and Patient Outcomes.*Annals of Surgery*. 2014;259(6):1041-1053. doi:10.1097/SLA.0000000000000595.

6. West, C. P., Shanafelt, T. D., & Kolars, J. C. (2011). Quality of life, burnout, educational debt, and medical knowledge among internal medicine residents. *JAMA*, *306*(9), 952-960.

7. Thomas, N. K. (2004). Resident burnout. *JAMA, 292*(23), 2880-2889.

8. Chen, P. W. (October 1, 2009). When the Doctor Is Distressed. *The New York Times*. Accessed on 10-4-2017 from http://www.nytimes.com/2009/10/01/health/01chen.html.

9. Papadakis, M. A., Paauw, D. S., Hafferty, F. W., Shapiro, J., Byyny, R. L., & Alpha Omega Alpha Honor Medical Society Think Tank. (2012). Perspective: the education community must develop best practices informed by evidence-based research to remediate lapses of professionalism. *Academic Medicine*,*87*(12), 1694-1698.

10. Dunn, P. M., Arnetz, B. B., Christensen, J. F., & Homer, L. (2007). Meeting the imperative to improve physician well-being: assessment of an innovative program.*Journal of general internal medicine*,*22*(11), 1544-1552.

11. McPhee, S. J., & Rabow, M. W. Doctoring to Heal: fostering well-being among physicians through personal reflection.*Western Journal of Medicine*,*1*(174), 66-69.

12. Mushin, I. C., Matteson, M. T., & Lynch, E. C. (1993). Developing a resident assistance program: beyond the support group model.*Archives of internal medicine*,*153*(6), 729-733.

13. Levinson, W., Ginsburg, S., Hafferty, F., & Lucey, C. R. (2014).*Understanding medical professionalism*. McGraw Hill Professional.

14. Frei, E., Stamm, M., & Buddeberg-Fischer, B. (2010). Mentoring programs for medical students-a review of the PubMed literature 2000-2008.*BMC medical education*,*10*(1), 32.

15. Frei, E., Stamm, M., & Buddeberg-Fischer, B. (2010). Mentoring programs for medical students-a review of the PubMed literature 2000-2008.*BMC medical education*,*10*(1), 32.

16. Sambunjak, D., Straus, S. E., & Marusic, A. (2010). A systematic review of qualitative research on the meaning and characteristics of mentoring in academic medicine.*Journal of general internal medicine,25*(1), 72-78.

17. Shanafelt, T. D., Dyrbye, L. N., & West, C. P. (2017). Addressing Physician Burnout: The Way Forward. *Jama,317*(9), 901-902.

18. Ivancevich, J. M., Matteson, M. T., & Konopaske, R. (1990). Organizational behavior and management.

19. Matteson, M. T., & Ivancevich, J. M. (1987).*Controlling work stress: Effective human resource and management strategies.* Jossey-Bass.

20. Eckleberry-Hunt, J., Van Dyke, A., Lick, D., & Tucciarone, J. (2009). Changing the conversation from burnout to wellness: physician well-being in residency training programs. *Journal of graduate medical education,1*(2), 225-230.

21. Levey, R. E. (2001). Sources of stress for residents and recommendations for programs to assist them. *Academic Medicine,76*(2), 142-150.

22. Satterfield, J. M., & Becerra, C. (2010). Faculty and student support: developmental challenges, stressors and coping strategies in medical residents: a qualitative analysis of support groups. *Medical education,44*(9), 908-916.

23. Wright, S. M., Levine, R. B., Beasley, B., Haidet, P., Gress, T. W., Caccamese, S., ... & Kern, D. E. (2006). Personal growth and its correlates during residency training.*Medical education,40*(8), 737-745.

24. McKevitt, C., Morgan, M., Dundas, R., & Holland, W. W. (1997). Sickness absence and 'working through' illness: a comparison of two professional groups. *Journal of Public Health, 19*(3), 295-300.

25. Thompson, W. T., Cupples, M. E., Sibbett, C. H., Skan, D. I., & Bradley, T. (2001). Challenge of culture, conscience, and contract to general practitioners' care of their own health: qualitative study. *BMJ: British Medical Journal, 323*(7315), 728.

26. Uallachain, G. N. (2007). Attitudes towards self-health care: a survey of GP trainees. *Irish Medical Journal, 100*(6), 489-491.

27. Davis, M., Detre, T., Ford, D. E., Hansbrough, W., Hendin, H., Laszlo, J., ... & Silverman, M. M. (2003). Confronting depression and suicide in physicians: a consensus statement. *JAMA, 289*(23), 3161-3166.

28. Worley, L. L. (2008). Our fallen peers: a mandate for change. *Academic Psychiatry, 32*(1), 8-12.

29. Schroeder, R., Brazeau, C. M., Zackin, F., Rovi, S., Dickey, J., Johnson, M. S., & Keller, S. E. (2009). Do state medical board applications violate the Americans with Disabilities Act? *Academic Medicine, 84*(6), 776-781.

30. Hampton, T. (2005). Experts address risk of physician suicide. *JAMA, 294*(10), 1189-1191.

CHAPTER 4:

1. Shanafelt, T. D., Dyrbye, L. N., & West, C. P. (2017). Addressing Physician Burnout: The Way Forward. *Jama,317*(9), 901-902.

CHAPTER 5:

1. Mushin, I. C., Matteson, M. T., & Lynch, E. C. (1993). Developing a resident assistance program: beyond the support group model.*Archives of internal medicine,153*(6), 729-733.

2. Ivancevich, J. M., Matteson, M. T., & Konopaske, R. (1990). Organizational behavior and management.

3. Matteson, M. T., & Ivancevich, J. M. (1987).*Controlling work stress: Effective human resource and management strategies.* Jossey-Bass.

4. American Academy of Family Physicians (1979). Coping: Stress and the Resident Physician. Kansas City, Mo.

CHAPTER 6:

1. [online] Available at: https://www.stepsforward.org/ [Accessed 9 Oct. 2017].

2. Ivancevich, J. M., Matteson, M. T., & Konopaske, R. (1990). Organizational behavior and management.

3. Kaye, A. D., Okanlawon, O. J., & Urman, R. D. (2014). Clinical performance feedback and quality improvement opportunities for perioperative physicians.*Advances in medical education and practice,5*, 115.

4. O'Daniel, M., & Rosenstein, A. H. (2008). Professional communication and team collaboration, Ch. 33.

5. Weller, J., Boyd, M., & Cumin, D. (2014). Teams, tribes and patient safety: overcoming barriers to effective teamwork in healthcare.*Postgraduate medical journal,90*(1061), 149-154.

6. Taran, S. (2011). An examination of the factors contributing to poor communication outside the physician-patient sphere.*McGill Journal of Medicine: MJM,13*(1).

7. Weller, J. M., Barrow, M., & Gasquoine, S. (2011). Interprofessional collaboration among junior doctors and nurses in the hospital setting.*Medical education,45*(5), 478-487.

8. Levinson, W., Ginsburg, S., Hafferty, F., & Lucey, C. R. (2014).*Understanding medical professionalism.* McGraw Hill Professional, Ch. 12.

CHAPTER 7:

1. Yao DC, Wright SM. The Challenge of Problem Residents.*Journal of General Internal Medicine.* 2001;16(7):486-492. doi:10.1046/j.1525-1497.2001.016007486.x.

2. Dyrbye, L. N., West, C. P., Sinsky, C. A., Goeders, L. E., Satele, D. V., & Shanafelt, T. D. (2017, October). Medical Licensure Questions and Physician Reluctance to Seek Care for Mental Health Conditions. In*Mayo Clinic Proceedings*(Vol. 92, No. 10, pp. 1486-1493). Elsevier.

3. Bangal, V. B., Shinde, K. K., & Gavhane, S. P. (2012). STRESS AT THE WORKPLACE DURING RESIDENCY TRAINING.*International Journal of Biomedical Research,3*(9), 381-385.

4. Matteson, M. T., & Ivancevich, J. M. (1987).*Controlling work stress: Effective human resource and management strategies.* Jossey-Bass.

5. Ivancevich, J. M., Matteson, M. T., & Konopaske, R. (1990). Organizational behavior and management.

6. Howell, J. B., & Schroeder, D. P. (1984).*Physician stress: a handbook for coping.* University Park Press.

CHAPTER 8:

1. Casalino, L. P., & Crosson, F. J. (2015). Physician Satisfaction and Physician Well-Being: Should Anyone Care?.*Professions and Professionalism*,*5*(1).

2. Papadakis, M. A., Hodgson, C. S., Teherani, A., & Kohatsu, N. D. (2004). Unprofessional behavior in medical school is associated with subsequent disciplinary action by a state medical board.*Academic Medicine*,*79*(3), 244-249.

3. Papadakis, M. A., Teherani, A., Banach, M. A., Knettler, T. R., Rattner, S. L., Stern, D. T., ... & Hodgson, C. S. (2005). Disciplinary action by medical boards and prior behavior in medical school. *New England Journal of Medicine*,*353*(25), 2673-2682.

4. Egener, B. E., Mason, D. J., McDonald, W. J., Okun, S., Gaines, M. E., Fleming, D. A., ... & Andresen, M. L. (2017). The charter on professionalism for health care organizations.*Academic Medicine*,*92*(8), 1091.

5. Egener, B., McDonald, W., Rosof, B., & Gullen, D. (2012). Perspective: organizational professionalism: relevant competencies and behaviors.*Academic Medicine*,*87*(5), 668-674.

6. Cruess, S. R., & Cruess, R. L. (2008). Understanding medical professionalism: a plea for an inclusive and integrated approach.*Medical education*,*42*(8), 755-757.

7. Anderson, R. A., & McDaniel Jr, R. R. (2000). Managing health care organizations: where professionalism meets complexity science.*Health care management review*,*25*(1), 83-92.

8. Shapiro, J., Whittemore, A., & Tsen, L. C. (2014). Instituting a culture of professionalism: the establishment of a center for professionalism and peer support.*The Joint Commission Journal on Quality and Patient Safety*,*40*(4), 168-AP1.

9. Cunningham, A. T., Bernabeo, E. C., Wolfson, D. B., & Lesser, C. S. (2011). Organisational strategies to cultivate professional values and behaviours.*Quality and Safety in Health Care*, bmjqs-2010.

10. Daugherty, S. R., Baldwin Jr, D. C., & Rowley, B. D. (1998). Learning, satisfaction, and mistreatment during medical internship: a national survey of working conditions.*JAMA*,*279*(15), 1194-1199.

11. Leisy, H. B., & Ahmad, M. (2016). Altering workplace attitudes for resident education (AWARE): discovering solutions for medical resident bullying through literature review.*BMC medical education*,*16*(1), 127.

12. Papadakis, M. A., Loeser, H., & Healy, K. (2001). Early detection and evaluation of professionalism deficiencies in medical students: one school's approach.*Academic medicine*,*76*(11), 1100-1106.

CHAPTER 9:

1. Young, J. Q., Ranji, S. R., Wachter, R. M., Lee, C. M., Niehaus, B., & Auerbach, A. D. (2011). "July effect": impact of the academic year-end changeover on patient outcomes: a systematic review.*Annals of internal medicine*,*155*(5), 309-315.

2. Hughes, E. "July Effect? Maybe Not." *Canadian Medical Association Journal*, August 14, 2017,vol. 189,no. 32.

3. Myers, L., Mikhael, B., Currier, P., Berg, K., Jena, A., Donnino, M., ... & American Heart Association's Get with the Guidelines-Resuscitation Investigators. (2017). The association between physician turnover (the "July Effect") and survival after in-hospital cardiac arrest.*Resuscitation*,*114*, 133-140.

4. Shah, A. Y., Abreo, A., Akar-Ghibril, N., Cady, R. F., & Shah, R. K. (2017). Is the "July Effect" Real? Pediatric Trainee Reported Medical Errors and Adverse Events.*Pediatric Quality & Safety*,*2*(2), e018.

5. Shah, A. A., Zogg, C. K., Nitzschke, S. L., Changoor, N. R., Havens, J. M., Salim, A., ... & Haider, A. H. (2016). Evaluation of the perceived association between resident turnover and the outcomes of patients who undergo emergency general surgery: questioning the July phenomenon.*JAMA surgery,151*(3), 217-224.

6. Haller, G., Myles, P. S., Taffé, P., Perneger, T. V., & Wu, C. L. (2009). Rate of undesirable events at beginning of academic year: retrospective cohort study.*Bmj,339*, b3974.

7. Wei, E. K., Sarff, L., & Spellberg, B. (2017). Debunking the July Effect Myth.*Journal of patient safety.*

8. Burke, L. G., Frakt, A. B., Khullar, D., Orav, E. J., & Jha, A. K. (2017). Association Between Teaching Status and Mortality in US Hospitals.*Jama,317*(20), 2105-2113.

9. Kirchheimer, S. (Updated 2013, June). Medical Errors Increase in Hospitals in July - July Effect. Retrieved October 11, 2017, from http://www.aarp.org/health/doctors-hospitals/info-06-2010/why_you_should_avoid_the_hospital_in_july.html

10. Neale, A. V., Bowman, M. A., & Seehusen, D. A. (2017). Improving family medicine with thoughtful research.*The Journal of the American Board of Family Medicine,30*(2), 117-120.

11. Mims, L. D., Porter, M., Simpson, K. N., & Carek, P. J. (2017). The "July Effect": A Look at July Medical Admissions in Teaching Hospitals.*The Journal of the American Board of Family Medicine,30*(2), 189-195.

12. Pettit, J. E. (2015). Coleadership among chief residents: exploration of experiences across specialties. *Journal of graduate medical education,7*(2), 203-207.

13. Antonoff, M. B., Swanson, J. A., Acton, R. D., Chipman, J. G., Maddaus, M. A., Schmitz, C. C., & D'cunha, J. (2010). Improving surgery intern confidence through the implementation of expanded orientation sessions. *Surgery, 148*(2), 181-186.

14. Taitz, J., Brydon, M., & Duffy, D. (2004). Making the Most of Medical Orientation—A New Approach. *Medical Education Online,9*(1), 4361.

15. Matteson, M. T., & Ivancevich, J. M. (1987).*Controlling work stress: Effective human resource and management strategies.* Jossey-Bass.

CHAPTER 10:

1. Schlosser, B., M.D., Ph.D. (n.d.). Do more with the time you have: 13 time management tips for harried residents.*American Academy of Dermatology Association.* Retrieved October 11, 2017, from https://www.aad.org/members/publications/directions-in-residency/archivee-time-you-have-13-time-management-tips-for-harried-residents

2. Abdellatif, A., Bagian, J. P., Barajas, E. R., Cohen, M., Cousins, D., Denham, C. R., ... & Horvath, D. (2007). Communication During Patient Hand-Overs.*Joint Commission Journal on Quality and Patient Safety,33*(7), 439-442.

3. *Staying mindful: Time management tips for residents*[Pdf]. (n.d.). Royal College of Physicians and Surgeons of Canada.

4. Levine, B. (1970, January 01). Time Management. Retrieved October 11, 2017, from http://www.americanresidentproject.net/blog/time-management. The American Resident Project.

5. Young, J. Q., Ranji, S. R., Wachter, R. M., Lee, C. M., Niehaus, B., & Auerbach, A. D. (2011). "July effect": impact of the academic year-end changeover on patient outcomes: a systematic review.*Annals of internal medicine,155*(5), 309-315.

6. Anderson, J. G. (2004). Surgical Training, Error.*Jama,291*(14), 1775-1776.

7. Makary, M. A., & Daniel, M. (2016). Medical error-the third leading cause of death in the US.*BMJ: British Medical Journal (Online),353*.

CHAPTER 11:

1. Yuen, J. K., Reid, M. C., & Fetters, M. D. (2011). Hospital do-not-resuscitate orders: why they have failed and how to fix them.*Journal of general internal medicine,26*(7), 791-797.

2. Chung H-O, Oczkowski SJW, Hanvey L, Mbuagbaw L, You JJ. Educational interventions to train health care professionals in end-of-life communication: a systematic review and meta-analysis.*BMC Medical Education.* 2016; 16:131. doi: 10.1186/s12909-016-0653-x.

3. Workman, S. (2007). A communication model for encouraging optimal care at the end of life for hospitalized patients.*Qjm,100*(12), 791-797.

4. Vozenilek, J., Huff, J. S., Reznek, M., & Gordon, J. A. (2004). See one, do one, teach one: advanced technology in medical education.*Academic Emergency Medicine,11*(11), 1149-1154.

5. Oncotalk: Improving Oncologists' Communication Skills. (n.d.). Retrieved October 11, 2017, from http://depts.washington.edu/oncotalk/learn/modules.html

6. Woo, J. A., Maytal, G., & Stern, T. A. (2006). Clinical challenges to the delivery of end-of-life care. *Primary care companion to the journal of clinical psychiatry,8*(6), 367.

7. Einstein, D. J., Einstein, K. L., & Mathew, P. (2015). Dying for advice: code status discussions between resident physicians and patients with advanced cancer—a national survey.*Journal of palliative medicine,18*(6), 535-541.

8. Szmuilowicz E, Neely KJ, Sharma RK, Cohen ER, McGaghie WC, Wayne DB. Improving Residents' Code Status Discussion Skills: A Randomized Trial.*Journal of Palliative Medicine.* 2012;15(7):768-774. doi:10.1089/jpm.2011.0446.

9. Anderson WG, Chase R, Pantilat SZ, Tulsky JA, Auerbach AD. Code Status Discussions Between Attending Hospitalist Physicians and Medical Patients at Hospital Admission.*Journal of General Internal Medicine.* 2011; 26(4):359-366. doi:10.1007/s11606-010-1568-6.

10. Kagawa-Singer, M., & Blackhall, L. J. (2001). Negotiating cross-cultural issues at the end of life: you got to go where he lives.*Jama,286*(23), 2993-3001.

11. Park, E. R., Betancourt, J. R., Miller, E., Nathan, M., MacDonald, E., Ananeh-Firempong, O., & Stone, V. E. (2006). Internal Medicine Residents' Perceptions of Cross-Cultural Training.*Journal of general internal medicine,21*(5), 476-480.

12. Gawande, A. (2014).*Being mortal: medicine and what matters in the end.* Macmillan.

13. Sulmasy, D. P., & Snyder, L. (2010). Substituted interests and best judgments: an integrated model of surrogate decision making.*JAMA,304*(17), 1946-1947.

14. Teno, J. M., Gruneir, A., Schwartz, Z., Nanda, A., & Wetle, T. (2007). Association between advance directives and quality of end-of-life care: A national study.*Journal of the American Geriatrics Society,55*(2), 189-194.

15. Wissow, L. S., Belote, A., Kramer, W., Compton-Phillips, A., Kritzler, R., & Weiner, J. P. (2004). Promoting advance directives among elderly primary care patients.*Journal of general internal medicine,19*(9), 944-951.

16. Kyle P. Edmonds, MD, Palliative Physician | Quality Medical Director | Educator | Leader Follow. (2013, November 21). The "Code Status" Conversation. Retrieved October 11, 2017, from https://www.slideshare.net/KylePEdmondsMD/code-status

17. Anderson, W. G., Chase, R., Pantilat, S. Z., Tulsky, J. A., & Auerbach, A. D. (2011). Code status discussions between attending hospitalist physicians and medical patients at hospital admission. *Journal of general internal medicine,26*(4), 359-366.

18. Lo, B, & Tulsky, J.A.. (July 2003). Code Status Confusion, Agency for Healthcare Research and Quality , https://psnet.ahrq.gov/webmm/case/25/code-status-confusion

19. Silveira, M. J., Kim, S. Y., & Langa, K. M. (2010). Advance directives and outcomes of surrogate decision making before death.*New England Journal of Medicine,362*(13), 1211-1218.

CHAPTER 12:

1. Levetown, M. (2008). Communicating with children and families: from everyday interactions to skill in conveying distressing information.*Pediatrics,121*(5), e1441-e1460.

2. Mitnick, S., Leffler, C., Hood, V. L., & American College of Physicians Ethics, Professionalism and Human Rights Committee. (2010). Family caregivers, patients and physicians: ethical guidance to optimize relationships.*Journal of general internal medicine,25*(3), 255-260.

3. *Caregiving in the U.S.*[Pdf]. (2015, June). Conducted for National Alliance for Caregiving and the AARP Public Policy Institute by Greenwald & Associates.

4. Berman, E. M., Heru, A., Grunebaum, H., Rolland, J., Sargent, J., Wamboldt, M., ... & Group for the Advancement of Psychiatry Committee on the Family. (2008). Family-oriented patient care through the residency training cycle.*Academic Psychiatry,32*(2), 111-118.

5. Clay, A. M., & Parsh, B. (2016). Patient-and family-centered care: It's not just for pediatrics anymore. *AMA journal of ethics,18*(1), 40.

6. Bertakis, K. D., & Azari, R. (2011). Patient-centered care is associated with decreased health care utilization.*The Journal of the American Board of Family Medicine,24*(3), 229-239.

7. Schleiter, K. E. (2009). Difficult patient-physician relationships and the risk of medical malpractice litigation.*Virtual Mentor,11*(3), 242.

8. Vincent, C., Phillips, A., & Young, M. (1994). Why do people sue doctors? A study of patients and relatives taking legal action.*The Lancet,343*(8913), 1609-1613.

9. Beckman, H. B., Markakis, K. M., Suchman, A. L., & Frankel, R. M. (1994). The doctor-patient relationship and malpractice: lessons from plaintiff depositions.*Archives of internal medicine,154*(12), 1365-1370.

10. Back, A. L., & Arnold, R. M. (2005). Dealing with conflict in caring for the seriously ill:"it was just out of the question".*Jama,293*(11), 1374-1381.

11. Bloche, M. G. (2005). Managing conflict at the end of life.*New England Journal of Medicine,352*(23), 2371-2373.

12. *Communication skills education for doctors: An update* [Pdf]. (2004). British Medical Assoication.

13. Ha, J. F., & Longnecker, N. (2010). Doctor-patient communication: a review.*The Ochsner Journal,10*(1), 38-43.

14. Ranjan, P., Kumari, A., & Chakrawarty, A. (2015). How can doctors improve their communication skills?.*Journal of clinical and diagnostic research: JCDR,9*(3), JE01.

15. Bevans, M., & Sternberg, E. M. (2012). Caregiving burden, stress, and health effects among family caregivers of adult cancer patients.*Jama,307*(4), 398-403.

16. Feldman, H. M., Ploof, D., & Cohen, W. I. (1999). Physician-family partnerships: the adaptive practice model.*Journal of Developmental & Behavioral Pediatrics,20*(2), 111-116.

17. Weitzman, P. F., & Weitzman, E. A. (2003). Promoting communication with older adults: protocols for resolving interpersonal conflicts and for enhancing interactions with doctors.*Clinical Psychology Review,23*(4), 523-535.

18. Hoppe, R. B., King, A. M., Mazor, K. M., Furman, G. E., Wick-Garcia, P., Corcoran–Ponisciak, H., & Katsufrakis, P. J. (2013). Enhancement of the assessment of physician–patient communication skills in the United States medical licensing examination.*Academic Medicine,88*(11), 1670-1675.

CHAPTER 13

1. Sabherwal, N., Mittal, A., Pandey, N.K., Kanshal, G., Kaustav, P. (2015). A study of Patient Physician Communication and Barriers in Communication. [Pdf]. International Journal of Research Foundation of Hospital & Health care Administration.

2. Levinson, W. (1994). Physician-patient communication: a key to malpractice prevention.*Jama,272*(20), 1619-1620.

3. Schleiter, K. E. (2009). Difficult patient-physician relationships and the risk of medical malpractice litigation.*Virtual Mentor,11*(3), 242.

4. Haas, L. J., Leiser, J. P., Magill, M. K., & Sanyer, O. N. (2005). Management of the difficult patient. *Am Fam Physician,72*(10), 2063-8.

5. Derksen, F., Bensing, J., & Lagro-Janssen, A. (2013). Effectiveness of empathy in general practice: a systematic review.*Br J Gen Pract,63*(606), e76-e84.

6. Hull, S. K., & Broquet, K. (2007). How to manage difficult patient encounters.*Family practice management,14*(6), 30.

7. Steinmetz, D., & Tabenkin, H. (2001). The 'difficult patient' as perceived by family physicians.*Family practice,18*(5), 495-500.

8. Hahn, S. R., Kroenke, K., Spitzer, R. L., Brody, D., Williams, J. B., Linzer, M., & Verloin deGruy, F. (1996). The difficult patient.*Journal of general internal medicine,11*(1), 1-8.

9. Groves, J. (2009). Taking care of the hateful patient.*Personality Disorder the Definitive Reader,* 52-63.

10. Zolnierek, K. B. H., & DiMatteo, M. R. (2009). Physician communication and patient adherence to treatment: a meta-analysis.*Medical care,47*(8), 826.

11. Ofri, D. (June 4, 2013). The Darkest Year of Medical School. *Medical Examiner.*

12. Levinson, W., Lesser, C. S., & Epstein, R. M. (2010). Developing physician communication skills for patient-centered care.*Health affairs,29*(7), 1310-1318.

13. Atluru, A. (2016, August 24). What Improv Can Teach Tomorrow's Doctors. Retrieved October 11, 2017, from https://www.theatlantic.com/education/archive/2016/08/what-improv-can-teach-tomorrows-doctors/497177/

14. Pomm, H. A., Shahady, E., & Pomm, R. M. (2004). The CALMER approach: Teaching learners six steps to serenity when dealing with difficult patients. *FAMILY MEDICINE-KANSAS CITY-,36*(7), 467-469.

15. Jackson, J. L., & Kroenke, K. (1999). Difficult patient encounters in the ambulatory clinic: clinical predictors and outcomes. *Archives of Internal Medicine,159*(10), 1069-1075.

16. Ha, J. F., & Longnecker, N. (2010). Doctor-patient communication: a review. *The Ochsner Journal,10*(1), 38-43.

17. Drossman, D. A. (2013). 2012 David Sun lecture: helping your patient by helping yourself--how to improve the patient-physician relationship by optimizing communication skills. *The American journal of gastroenterology,108*(4), 521.

18. Barry, C. A., Bradley, C. P., Britten, N., Stevenson, F. A., & Barber, N. (2000). Patients' unvoiced agendas in general practice consultations: qualitative study. *Bmj,320*(7244), 1246-1250.

19. Hoppe, R. B., King, A. M., Mazor, K. M., Furman, G. E., Wick-Garcia, P., Corcoran–Ponisciak, H., & Katsufrakis, P. J. (2013). Enhancement of the assessment of physician–patient communication skills in the United States medical licensing examination. *Academic Medicine,88*(11), 1670-1675.

CHAPTER 14:

1. Narayanan, V., Bista, B., & Koshy, C. (2010). 'BREAKS'protocol for breaking bad news. *Indian journal of palliative care,16*(2), 61.

2. Fallowfield, L., & Jenkins, V. (2004). Communicating sad, bad, and difficult news in medicine. *The Lancet,363*(9405), 312-319.

3. Vandekieft, G. K. (2001). Breaking bad news. *American family physician,64*(12).

4. Thornton, J. D., Pham, K., Engelberg, R. A., Jackson, J. C., & Curtis, J. R. (2009). Families with limited English proficiency receive less information and support in interpreted ICU family conferences. *Critical care medicine,37*(1), 89.

5. Juckett, G., & Unger, K. (2014). Appropriate use of medical interpreters. *American family physician,90*(7).

6. Hagerty, R. G., Butow, P. N., Ellis, P. M., Lobb, E. A., Pendlebury, S. C., Leighl, N., ... & Tattersall, M. H. (2005). Communicating with realism and hope: incurable cancer patients' views on the disclosure of prognosis. *Journal of clinical oncology,23*(6), 1278-1288.

7. Fischer, G. S., & Arnold, R. M. (2007). Feasibility of a brief workshop on palliative care communication skills for medical interns. *Journal of palliative medicine,10*(1), 19-23.

8. Arnold, R. (2005). *Empathic intelligence: Teaching, learning, relating.* UNSW Press.

9. Neumann, M., Edelhäuser, F., Tauschel, D., Fischer, M. R., Wirtz, M., Woopen, C., ... & Scheffer, C. (2011). Empathy decline and its reasons: a systematic review of studies with medical students and residents. *Academic medicine,86*(8), 996-1009.

10. Minichiello, T. A., Ling, D., & Ucci, D. K. (2007). Breaking bad news: a practical approach for the hospitalist. *Journal of hospital medicine,2*(6), 415-421.

11. Back, A. L., Arnold, R. M., Baile, W. F., Fryer-Edwards, K. A., Alexander, S. C., Barley, G. E., ... & Tulsky, J. A. (2007). Efficacy of communication skills training for giving bad news and discussing transitions to palliative care. *Archives of internal medicine,167*(5), 453-460.

12. Back, A. L., Arnold, R. M., Baile, W. F., Tulsky, J. A., & Fryer-Edwards, K. (2005). Approaching difficult communication tasks in oncology.*CA: A Cancer Journal for Clinicians,55*(3), 164-177.

13. Whitney, S. N., McCullough, L. B., Frugé, E., McGuire, A. L., & Volk, R. J. (2008). Beyond breaking bad news.*Cancer,113*(2), 442-445.

CHAPTER 15:

1. Goodall, A. H., Stoller, J. K., & Bäker, A. (2016). Why The Best Hospitals Are Managed by Doctors. *Harvard Business Review.*

2. Accreditation Council for Graduate Medical Education. (n.d.). Retrieved November 07, 2017, from http://www.acgme.org/

3. Nguyen, H. H. (2010). Hospitalist to home: outpatient parenteral antimicrobial therapy at an academic center.*Clinical Infectious Diseases,51*(Supplement_2), S220-S223.

4. Waldman, J. D., Smith, H. L., Hood, J. N., & Pappelbaum, S. J. (2006). Healthcare CEOs and physicians: reaching common ground/practitioner application.*Journal of healthcare management,51*(3), 171.

5. Nasca, T. J., Weiss, K. B., & Bagian, J. P. (2014). Improving clinical learning environments for tomorrow's physicians.*New England Journal of Medicine,370*(11), 991-993.

6. Kelley, C. A., & Brown, M. B. (1987). Quality circles in the hospital setting: their current status and potential for the future.*Health care management review,12*(1), 55-60.

CHAPTER 16:

1. Shanafelt, T. D., & Noseworthy, J. H. (2017, January). Executive leadership and physician well-being: nine organizational strategies to promote engagement and reduce burnout. In*Mayo Clinic Proceedings*(Vol. 92, No. 1, pp. 129-146). Elsevier.

2. Itani, K. M., Liscum, K., & Brunicardi, F. C. (2004). Physician leadership is a new mandate in surgical training.*The American journal of surgery,187*(3), 328-331.

3. Goleman, D. 2004. What makes a leader? (Best of HBR). Harvard Business Review, 82(1): 82–91.

4. Goleman, D., & Boyatzis, R. (2008). Social intelligence and the biology of leadership.*Harvard Business Review,86*(9), 74-81.

5. Salovey, P., & Mayer, J. D. (1990). Emotional intelligence. *Imagination, cognition and personality, 9*(3), 185-211.

6. Goleman, D. (1995). Emotional intelligence: Why it can matter more than IQ.

7. How Emotionally Intelligent Are You? (n.d.). Retrieved from http://thoughtpartnersinc.com/admin/uploads/howemotionallyintelligentareyoupdf.pdf Thought Partners Inc.

8. Jardine, D., Correa, R., Schultz, H., Nobis, A., Lanser, B. J., Ahmad, I., ... & Hinds, B. (2015). The need for a leadership curriculum for residents.

9. Goleman, D. (2000). Leadership that gets results.*Harvard business review,78*(2), 4-17.

10. Kong, F. J. (n.d.). Different styles of leadership. Retrieved October 11, 2017, from http://www.philstar.com/business/2012-09-30/854334/different-styles-leadership

CHAPTER 17:

1. Blumenthal, D. M., Bernard, K., Bohnen, J., & Bohmer, R. (2012). Addressing the leadership gap in medicine: residents' need for systematic leadership development training. *Academic Medicine,87*(4), 513-522.

2. Shanafelt, T. D., & Noseworthy, J. H. (2017, January). Executive leadership and physician well-being: nine organizational strategies to promote engagement and reduce burnout. In *Mayo Clinic Proceedings* (Vol. 92, No. 1, pp. 129-146). Elsevier.

3. Jardine, D., Correa, R., Schultz, H., Nobis, A., Lanser, B. J., Ahmad, I., ... & Hinds, B. (2015). The need for a leadership curriculum for residents.

4. Godbole, P., Burke, D., & Aylott, J. (Eds.). (2017). *Why Hospitals Fail: Between Theory and Practice.* Springer.

5. Weller, J., Boyd, M., & Cumin, D. (2014). Teams, tribes and patient safety: overcoming barriers to effective teamwork in healthcare. *Postgraduate medical journal,90*(1061), 149-154.

6. Mosser, G., & Begun, J. W. (2014). *Understanding teamwork in health care.* McGraw-Hill.

7. Hackman, J. R., Wageman, R., & Fisher, C. M. (2009). Leading teams when the time is right: Finding the best moments to act.

8. Lowe, J. I., & Herranen, M. (1982). Understanding teamwork: Another look at the concepts. *Social Work in Health Care,7*(2), 1-11.

9. Blumenthal, D. M., Bernard, K., Fraser, T. N., Bohnen, J., Zeidman, J., & Stone, V. E. (2014). Implementing a pilot leadership course for internal medicine residents: design considerations, participant impressions, and lessons learned. *BMC medical education,14*(1), 257.

10. Pediatrics in Practice. (n.d.). Retrieved October 11, 2017, from http://www.pediatricsinpractice.org/

11. Neher JO, Gordon KC, Meyer B, Stevens N. A five-step "microskills" model of clinical teaching. J Am Board Fam Pract. 1992 Jul-Aug;5(4):419-24.

12. UNC TeachingOnline.indd. (n.d.). Retrieved October 11, 2017, from https://www.med.unc.edu/pediatrics/education/teaching_center/monograph/MonographClinical.pdf

CHAPTER 19:

1. Lefebvre, D. C. (2012). Perspective: resident physician wellness: a new hope. *Academic medicine,87*(5), 598-602.

FACILITATOR MANUAL SAMPLE:

1. Burns, D. (2017, March 09). 014: The Five Secrets of Effective Communication (Part 1). Retrieved October 11, 2017, from https://feelinggood.com/2016/12/12/014-the-five-secrets-of-effective-communication-part-1/ https://feelinggood.com/2016/12/12/014-the-five-secrets-of-effective-communication-part-1/

2. Zastrow, C. (2011). *Brooks/Cole Empowerment Series: Social Work with Groups: A Comprehensive Workbook.* Nelson Education.

3. Zastrow, C., & Kirst-Ashman, K. (2006). *Understanding human behavior and the social environment.* Cengage Learning.

4. Howell, J. B., & Schroeder, D. P. (1984). *Physician stress: a handbook for coping.* University Park Press.

INDEX

CPSIA information can be obtained
at www.ICGtesting.com
Printed in the USA
BVHW02n1635080918
526927BV00003B/15/P